Hepatobiliary Medicine and Surgery - Gallbladder

Edited by Raimundas Lunevicius

Published in London, United Kingdom

Hepatobiliary Medicine and Surgery - Gallbladder
http://dx.doi.org/10.5772/intechopen.115525
Edited by Raimundas Lunevicius

Contributors
Aleksandar Zlatarov, Amit Gupta, Ammapalem Satish, Arunkumar V, Eirini Tsoutsou, Georgios Bointas, Indah Jamtani, Ioannis N. Gerogiannis, Karamveer Singh, Karl Heinz Leonhardt Rowika, Mark Sidhom, Mehrshad Ebrahimnezhad, Monisha Selvarasu, Nafilla Nesantya Sabatini, Prasoon Saxena, Raimundas Lunevicius, Razhan K. Ali, Satish Ammapalem, Sergey Yurievich Muraviev, Tsvetelina Teneva, Vania Myralda Giamour Marbun

First published in London, United Kingdom, 2025 by IntechOpen
IntechOpen is the global imprint of INTECHOPEN LIMITED, registered in England and Wales, registration number: 11086078, 167-169 Great Portland Street, London, W1W 5PF, United Kingdom

For EU product safety concerns: IN TECH d.o.o., Prolaz Marije Krucifikse Kozulić 3, 51000 Rijeka, Croatia, info@intechopen.com or visit our website at intechopen.com.

British Library Cataloguing-in-Publication Data
A catalogue record for this book is available from the British Library

Hepatobiliary Medicine and Surgery - Gallbladder
Edited by Raimundas Lunevicius
p. cm.
Print ISBN 978-1-83635-271-6
Online ISBN 978-1-83635-270-9
eBook (PDF) ISBN 978-1-83635-272-3

If disposing of this product, please recycle the paper responsibly.

Meet the editor

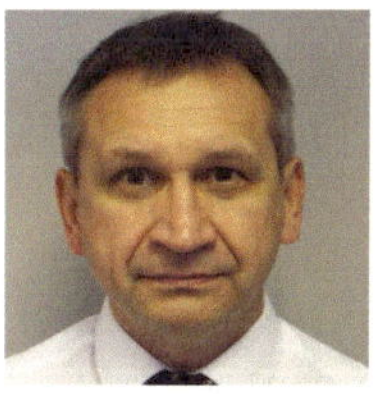

Raimundas Lunevicius, MD, Ph.D., DSc, FRCS, Professor, is a Consultant in Emergency General and Trauma Surgery at Aintree Hospital, NHS University Hospitals of Liverpool Group, UK, with extensive experience in biliary, gastrointestinal, abdominal wall, visceral trauma surgery, research, clinical audits, education, supervision, medical appraisal, academic editing, and review. He has completed three fellowship programmes: Monbushou (Nagoya University & Aichi Cancer Centre, Japan, 1998–2000), Fulbright–Humphrey (Johns Hopkins University, Bloomberg School of Public Health, US, 2008–2009), and King's College Hospital (2010–2012). His publications (h-index 78) include 263 refereed articles (PubMed 167), three monographs, seven book chapters, and three edited books (by 08-06-2025). He is the Editor-in-Chief of 'Emergency Care and Medicine' (MDPI, Switzerland) and a senior GBD Network collaborator (USA).

Contents

Preface

Since the launch of this open-access book project titled *Hepatobiliary Medicine and Surgery – Gallbladder* in November 2024, until its finalisation in June 2025, the project's aim has remained consistent: to share classical and contemporary knowledge about the gallbladder and its diseases from various perspectives in original and innovative ways. In total, 6 topics and 36 keywords have been selected to guide scientists, clinicians, researchers, educators, healthcare providers, and policymakers through the pre-planned structure of the book.

Emphasising the relationship between the gallbladder and biliary ductal system, along with other surrounding organs, anatomical structures, and tissues, is a crucial aspect of this undertaking. As gallstone disease and its management are among the predominant themes of this book, comprising seven chapters, it can be considered a continuation of the edited volume of *Gallstone Disease—Newer Insights and Current Trends*, published in 2024 (https://www.intechopen.com/books/12413).

This book possesses several unique characteristics, some of which merit mention. First, attention has been paid to the etymology of medical terms currently in use (*Anatomy of the Gallbladder* by I.N. Gerogiannis et al.). Second, new concepts such as asymptomatic cholecystitis (*Asymptomatic Cholecystitis: The Versatility of a Simple Clinical Question* by S.Y. Muraviev and M. Ebrahimnezhad), and three-layer, five-layer, or six-layer cholecystectomy are described. Third, with numerous original drawings and figures, this book is exceptionally well illustrated (e.g., *Imaging of Biliary Tree* by T. Teneva, A. Zlatarov, and the other chapters). Fourth, by employing Latin terms, this book emphasises the roots of modern medicine and medical ethics. Fifth, the relationship between anatomical details and surgical actions is highlighted in a new light (*Boon, Banes, and Cholecystectomy* by V.M.G. Marbun et al.). Sixth, readers will discover other details regarding the anatomy, physiology, and pathology of the gallbladder that are less frequently discussed among healthcare professionals, residents, and students in forums and scientific literature (*Mirizzi Syndrome and Its Management* by K. Singh et al., and other chapters). Seventh, this book details the patterns and levels of gallbladder wall thickening, based on its ultrasonographic intramural and extramural features, within the risk stratification framework known as the Gallbladder Reporting and Data System (*Gallbladder Carcinoma: A Comprehensive Review and Recent Updates* by A. Gupta et al.). Finally, the classification of cholecystectomies is emphasised, reminding readers that safety during gallbladder surgeries, as well as cultivating a culture of safety within the cholecystectomy surgical framework, are the top and primary priority (*Gallbladder and Bile Ducts: Anatomical Structures and Clinical Associations for 2025* by R. Lunevicius).

I want to express my gratitude to all the authors of the chapters for their valuable contributions to this project. Special thanks go to the IntechOpen staff, particularly Ms Nina Miocevic, the Publishing Process Manager, and Ms Sandra Bolf, the Senior Commissioning Editor.

I hope this open-access book, whether in its entirety or as individual chapters, will assist every reader in their ongoing studies of hepatobiliary medicine and surgery. Suggestions for improvement are welcome and will be taken into consideration.

Raimundas Lunevicius
Consultant Surgeon with Interest and Expertise in Hepatobiliary Surgery,
Department of General Emergency and Trauma Surgery,
Aintree Hospital,
NHS University Hospitals of Liverpool Group,
UK

Chapter 1

Anatomy of the Gallbladder

Ioannis N. Gerogiannis, Razhan K. Ali, Mark Sidhom, Georgios Bointas and Eirini Tsoutsou

Abstract

This chapter, Anatomy of the Gallbladder, serves as a foundational exploration of the gallbladder's structure, positioning, and physiological significance within the hepatobiliary system. It delves into the organ's gross anatomy, histological layers, vascular supply, lymphatic drainage, and innervation, highlighting its relationship with the liver, bile ducts, and surrounding structures. The chapter also examines anatomical variations and their clinical implications, offering insights into their relevance in surgical and diagnostic contexts. By providing a detailed overview, this section lays the groundwork for understanding gallbladder pathophysiology, disease management, and surgical interventions, positioning the reader to navigate subsequent topics in hepatobiliary medicine and surgery with a deeper anatomical perspective.

Keywords: gallbladder, anatomical variations, cystic artery, cystic duct, lymphatic drainage, gross anatomy

1. Introduction

The gallbladder is a relatively small organ located in the right upper quadrant of the abdomen. The gallbladder, which is pyriform in shape, is located in a fossa on the lower surface of the right lobe of the liver. It plays a crucial role in the digestive system by storing and concentrating the bile produced by the liver.

2. Orthographic origin and etymology

The term "gall bladder" is a compound noun formed within English by combining "gall" and "bladder." According to the Oxford English Dictionary (OED), the earliest recorded use of "gall bladder" dates back to 1676 in the writings of John Cooke [1].

The word "gall" originates from Old English "gealla," which is consistent with similar terms in other Germanic languages, such as Old Saxon "galia," Middle Dutch "galle," and Old High German "galla," all referring to bile.

The term "bladder" comes from Old English "blǣdre," meaning a blister or bladder, and is related to similar words in other Germanic languages.

Thus, "gall bladder" literally means "bile bladder," describing the organ's function as a storage sac for bile [1].

3. Embryology

The gallbladder arises from an endodermal outgrowth of the ventral side of the foregut at about the 4th week of embryonic life, together with the liver and bile ducts. This outgrowth appears as a cystic diverticulum just caudal to the newly formed hepatic duct and cephalad to the ventral pancreatic bud, just before the latter rotates to its dorsal position on the 32nd day. By day 35, the pedicle that connects the gallbladder to the hepatic duct is transformed into the cystic duct. In the 12th week, the production of bile begins, and the gallbladder and bile ducts become functional, storing the bile produced by the live (**Figure 1**) [2].

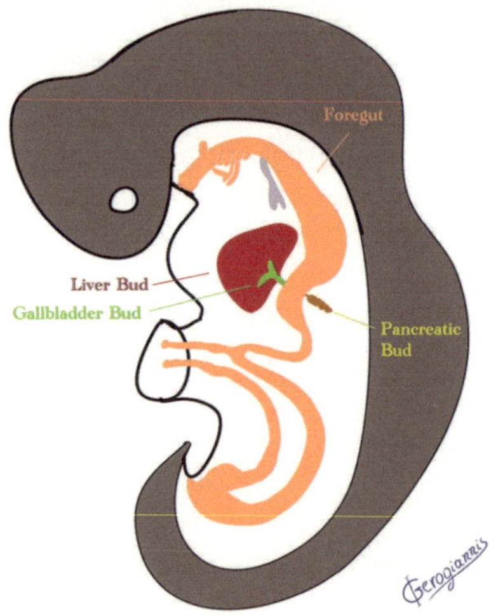

Figure 1.
Embryo (5th week of development). The gallbladder is present on the ventral side of the foregut, together with the liver and the hepatic duct. The pancreatic duct has already moved into its dorsal position.

4. Gross anatomy

4.1 Organ anatomy

The gallbladder is divided into three main sections:

i. *Fundus*: This is the rounded distal portion of the gallbladder, often extending beyond the inferior border of the liver. Clinically, the fundus is located at the level of the ninth costal cartilage, where the lateral edge of the right rectus abdominis muscle intersects the costal margin.

ii. *Body*: It is located between the fundus and the neck and is adjacent to the visceral surface of the liver.

iii. *Neck (infundibulum)*: This tapered segment connects the gallbladder to the cystic duct, which subsequently joins the common hepatic duct to form the common bile duct [3].

The *cystic duct* is a tube that connects the neck of the gallbladder to the common bile duct. It is typically 2–4 cm long and 2–3 mm in diameter, but this can vary [4]. However, it is difficult to predict the size of the lumen of the cystic duct. This is mainly because the mucosa of the lumen has multiple folds, making it appear as a spiral and tortuous tube. The spiral valve of Heister is a recognized block of valves made by the mucosal folds of the cystic duct together with smooth muscle fibers and a framework of connective tissue [3]. The role of the *Heister valves*, although several scientists have attempted to explain it, is not entirely clear; there may be an element of controlling the inflow outflow of the bile to and from the gallbladder, or/and the valves are just a development secondary to the evolution of the human adjusting to the erect posture [5]. Variations in the length and insertion of the cystic duct have been observed. It can range in length from 0.8 to 11.5 cm. In terms of insertion, the cystic duct can end in several places. The most frequent insertion is into the common hepatic duct, followed rarely by the right hepatic duct, the duodenum, and then the left hepatic duct [6].

Another anatomical entity evident in the majority of the population is the *Hartmann's pouch*. It presents as an outpouching of the gallbladder wall located in the area between the neck and the cystic duct. Finally, when the gallbladder is folded between the fundus and the neck, giving the appearance of a cap, it is called a *Phrygian cap*. This is seen in less than 6% of the general population and has no pathological significance (**Figure 2**) [7].

4.2 Location and topographic relations

The gallbladder is positioned in the right upper quadrant of the abdominal cavity. Its direction is oblique and therefore the fundus is more lateral and at a lower level than the neck, which is closer to the midline (**Figure 3**).

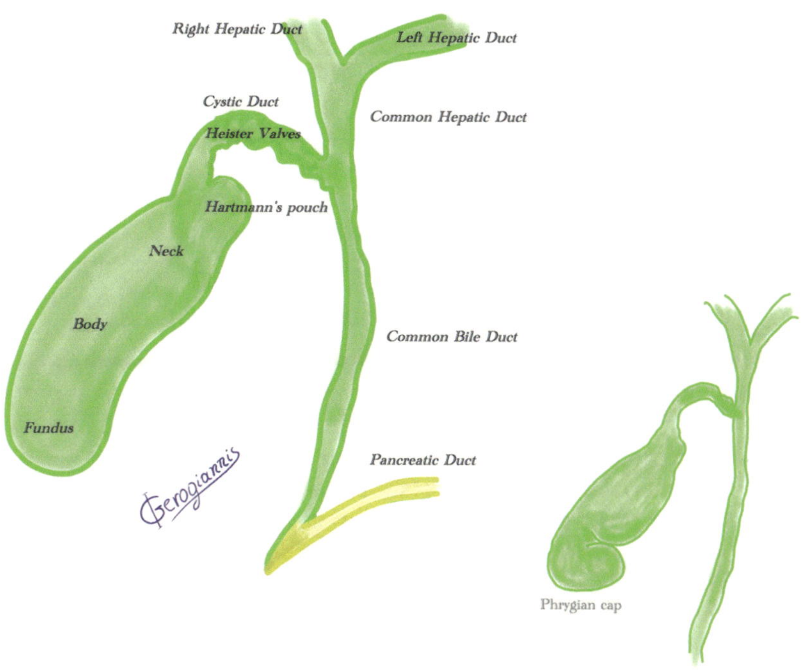

Figure 2.
Gross anatomy of the gallbladder and related ducts. Please note Hartmann's pouch and Heister valves. The Phrygian cap is also demonstrated.

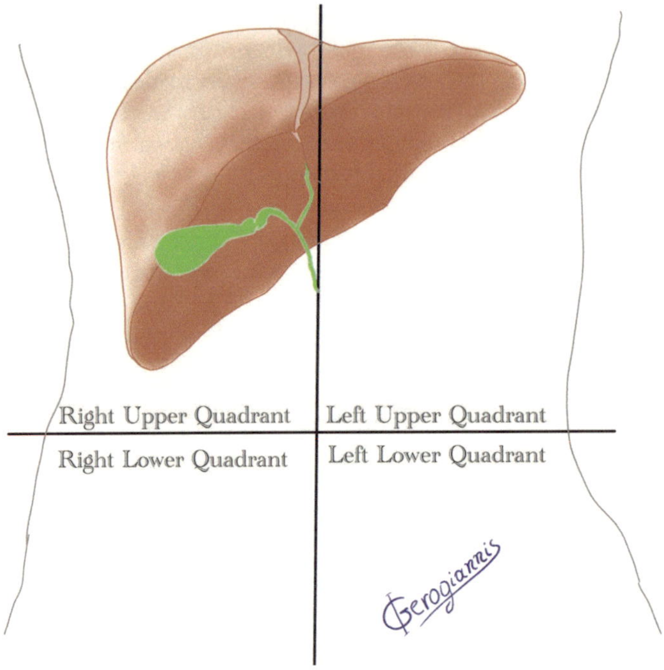

Figure 3.
Position of the gallbladder and its direction.

Except for the superior surface of its body, which attaches to the liver *via* areolar tissue, the gallbladder is generally covered by peritoneum. In some cases, the peritoneum fully surrounds the gallbladder, forming a short mesentery that attaches it to the liver.

The gallbladder maintains several important anatomical relationships:

Superiorly: It is in direct contact with the liver, specifically segments IVb and V [6]. Posteriorly: The gallbladder is related to the superior part of the duodenum, hepatic flexure, and the proximal transverse colon [3]. Inferiorly: It is adjacent to the transverse colon and, in some cases, the superior portion of the duodenum or the pyloric end of stomach [3].

More specifically, the fundus is completely covered by peritoneum and typically projects beyond the liver's sharp margin. Its anterior surface touches the peritoneum of the anterior abdominal wall, approximately where the transpyloric and midclavicular lines cross. Caudally, it lies above the right colic flexure and the proximal third of the transverse colon [3].

Cranially, the body of the gallbladder is attached to the liver while the rest of it is covered just with visceral peritoneum [3].

The neck of the gallbladder, like the body, is covered with visceral peritoneum in its majority, except the superior surface connects to the liver through loose areolar tissue containing the cystic artery and often a small lymphatic gland. Finally, inferiorly, it relates to the first part of the duodenum [3].

The cystic duct lies at the cranial part of the lesser omentum, and its course is above the first part of the duodenum. It also routes briefly parallel to and adheres to the postero-lateral aspect of the common hepatic duct.

The cystic artery is located parallel to the cystic duct, just cranial to it [3].

DOI: http://dx.doi.org/10.5772/intechopen.1011083

5. Vascular anatomy of the gallbladder

5.1 Arterial supply

5.1.1 The cystic artery and other branches

The cystic artery is the main arterial blood supply of the gallbladder. This typically arises from the right hepatic artery (**Figure 4**).

In most people, this artery passes through a small anatomic space called Calot's triangle—also known as the hepatobiliary triangle. The common hepatic duct, cystic duct, and inferior border of the liver form the boundaries of this triangle [8, 9].

The cystic artery usually divides into *superficial (anterior) and deep (posterior) branches. The superficial branch* provides blood supply to the peritoneal surface of the gallbladder while the deep *branch supplies the* hepatic surface of the gallbladder.

Small arterial branches may also arise from the cystic artery to supply blood to the cystic duct and adjacent bile ducts [10–13].

5.1.2 Variations in the cystic artery

Anatomic variations of the cystic artery are frequent, and incidences reported varied between 18.5% and 24.5% based on the population studied and imaging or dissection methods [12, 13]. Although the most frequent origin of the cystic artery

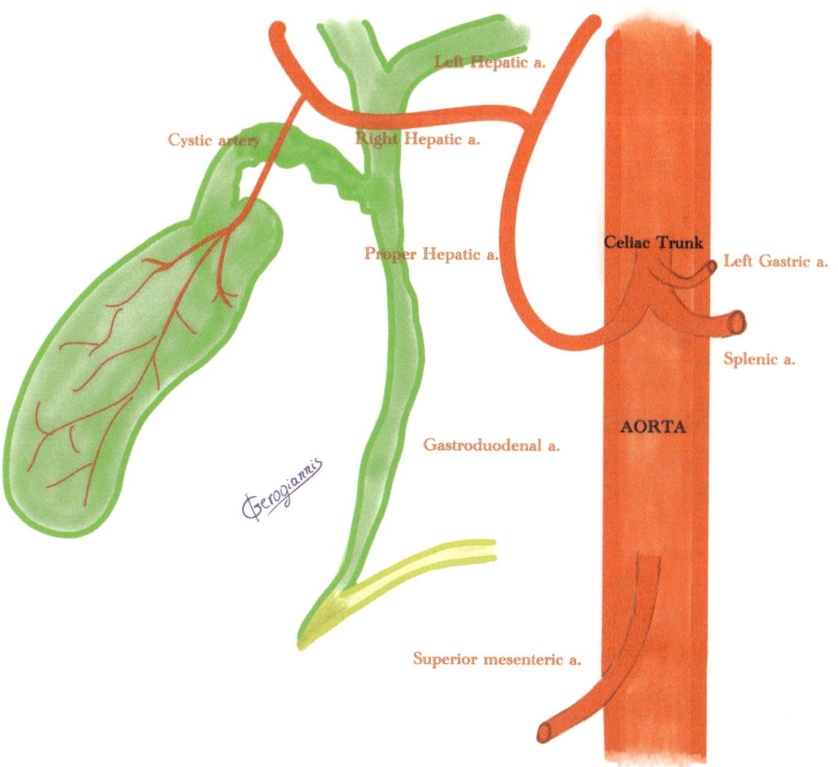

Figure 4.
Arterial supply of the gallbladder. a. corresponds to "artery."

is from the right hepatic artery, its origin, order of branching, and course may be changed because of embryological remodeling of the hepatic arterial tree [14].

5.1.2.1 Double cystic arteries

A "double" cystic artery arises when two distinct arteries supply the gallbladder, each coming from separate sources. Its incidence varies widely, reported from 2% up to 25% [14–15]. Recognizing this anomaly is crucial, as it can raise the risk of bleeding if unrecognized during surgery.

5.1.2.2 Aberrant origins of the cystic artery

1. *From the superior mesenteric artery*: Documented but rare [16].

2. *From the left hepatic artery*: Uncommon and can complicate dissection [17].

3. *From the common hepatic artery*: Risk of accidental ligation leading to hepatic ischemia [18].

4. *From the gastroduodenal artery*: Requires careful intraoperative identification [19].

5. *From the left gastric artery*: Extremely rare, though clinically relevant during procedures in the upper GI region [18].

5.1.2.3 Moynihan's hump

This variation describes a tortuous cystic artery that crosses over the common hepatic duct. It can be mistaken for the cystic duct, potentially causing ligation of the hepatic artery or bile ducts by accident [19].

5.1.2.4 Accessory cystic arteries

Small additional arteries may branch from the hepatic or gastroduodenal arteries. Missing one of these arteries during surgery can lead to unexpected bleeding if only the main cystic artery is ligated [20].

5.1.2.5 Course of the cystic artery

In some cases, the cystic artery passes either in front of or behind the common hepatic duct. This variation can increase the likelihood of misidentification or injury during gallbladder removal [21].

5.2 Venous drainage

Venous return from the gallbladder occurs through cystic veins, which typically follow two main pathways [8, 9]:

1. *Direct drainage into the liver parenchyma*: Small veins may flow directly into hepatic sinusoids rather than first entering the portal vein.

2. *Drainage into the portal system*: Cystic veins commonly drain into the portal vein (often its right branch) or small tributaries of the right portal vein.

Clinically, these routes are significant because they can serve as channels for gallbladder cancer to spread to the liver.

5.3 Lymphatic drainage

Lymphatic drainage from the gallbladder primarily goes to the cystic lymph node (often called the node of Lund), then to the hepatic and celiac lymph nodes. This pathway is important for understanding the potential spread of gallbladder tumors [8, 9].

6. Gallbladder innervation

6.1 Anterior hepatic plexus

The anterior hepatic plexus receives contributions from the *sympathetic and parasympathetic systems*. The *sympathetic fibers* derive from the celiac plexus, and the *parasympathetic fibers derive* primarily *via* the hepatic division of the anterior vagal trunk.

The pathway of the gallbladder's innervation starts with the hepatic branch of the anterior vagal trunk and travels through the hepatogastric ligament. Then, it joins the anterior hepatic plexus near the proper hepatic artery. From there, nerve branches accompany both superficial and deep branches of the cystic artery, reaching mainly the peritoneal aspect and the gallbladder bed.

The distribution of the nerves is primarily concentrated in the cystic duct and neck of the gallbladder, and fewer fibers extend toward the body and fundus. Notably, vagal branches do not directly reach the gallbladder independently but merge into the anterior hepatic plexus first [22].

6.2 Posterior hepatic plexus

The posterior hepatic plexus originates from the right side of the celiac plexus.

The pathway of the innervation starts and runs along the dorsal side of the portal vein. It is typically composed of four to five nerve fascicles divided into two bundles and predominantly accompanies the upper common bile duct and portal vein.

The Posterior Hepatic Plexus sends branches to gallbladder (primarily cystic duct and neck). It is also to the liver, the proximal descending duodenum, and the lower common bile duct.

It needs to be noted that the Posterior Hepatic Plexus shows abundant communication with the anterior hepatic plexus [22].

6.3 Phrenic nerves

The phrenic nerves derive mainly from the right phrenic nerve, occasionally from both right and left phrenic nerves. They are sometimes absent (in 20% of cases in Yi et al.'s study) [22].

The pathway of the innervation starts from the phrenic nerve branches that pass anteriorly toward the liver's hepatic portal, along the sagittal sulcus of the liver.

Their role likely includes sensory innervation contributing to referred pain in gallbladder pathology (shoulder-tip pain) [22].

7. Anatomical variations of the gallbladder

The gallbladder has several variations in its anatomy based on:

7.1 Morphological

The gallbladder exhibits various anatomical variations, both common and rare. One frequent variant is the Phrygian cap, where the fundus folds back on itself, which is important to recognize to avoid confusion. Another common variant is the sigmoid-shaped gallbladder. Less often, septations may occur, either congenital or resulting from chronic cholecystitis, and can be single or multiple. When numerous, these septations can create a characteristic "honeycomb" appearance.

Hartmann's pouch, also known as the infundibulum, refers to a localized outpouching near the gallbladder neck, adjacent to the body. This finding is often linked to cholelithiasis and may represent a pathological change rather than a normal anatomical variant. According to van Eijck et al. [23], Hartmann's pouch is considered a morphologic entity rather than a distinct anatomical structure [21]. A floating gallbladder, suspended by a peritoneal mesentery, is a rare variant that may increase the risk of torsion. Also uncommon are diverticula, which involve all layers of the gallbladder wall and should be differentiated from Rokitansky-Aschoff sinuses, which are mucosal outpouchings [24].

7.2 Congenital

7.2.1 Agenesis of the gallbladder

Gallbladder agenesis (GA) is a rare congenital anomaly where the gallbladder is completely absent, though the bile ducts remain normal. It is often discovered incidentally during surgery or autopsy, with most cases identified in patients around their mid-1940s. GA is more commonly seen in autopsy reports than surgical findings.

Gallbladder agenesis (GA) is often associated with other congenital abnormalities, affecting up to 30% of patients. These can involve multiple body systems, including the gastrointestinal, urinary, cardiovascular, and skeletal systems. Reported conditions include intestinal obstructions, abnormal intestinal positioning, kidney malformations, and limb anomalies such as fused fingers or toes, with genitourinary issues being particularly common.

While gallbladder agenesis (GA) typically occurs sporadically, there are cases where multiple family members are affected, hinting at a possible hereditary component. GA has also been linked to certain genetic syndromes, such as trisomy 18, and to prenatal exposure to teratogenic substances, like thalidomide [25].

7.2.2 Hypoplasia of the gallbladder

Hypoplastic gallbladder shares a similar etiology with gallbladder agenesis, in that the gallbladder bud is incompletely developed, or the solid primordium has failed to recanalize. Conditions like biliary atresia, chronic cholangitis, cystic fibrosis, and hepatitis in neonates are linked to this congenital anomaly. Approximately 33% of patients with a hypoplastic gallbladder experience symptoms, compared to 54% who remain asymptomatic. This rare condition should be considered when the gallbladder is not identified intraoperatively. Hypoplasia is less frequently reported than agenesis and is typically observed in children as a rudimentary structure, whereas in adults, it can result from post-inflammatory processes [26].

7.2.3 Duplication of the gallbladder

This anomaly occurs with an incidence of about 1 in 4000. However, the exact prevalence is difficult to determine, as it is typically only recognized in symptomatic cases or as incidental findings during laparotomy, imaging, or autopsy. There are two main types of gallbladder duplication described: (i) The Vesica fellea divisum or bi-lobed gallbladder and (ii) The Vesica fellea duplex or double gallbladder. In the Vesica fellea divisum, the lumen of the gallbladder is divided into two chambers, and embryologically, they share a common origin. In the Vesica fellea duplex, there is a dual embryological origin, and there are two gallbladders with their own cystic duct each. The differential diagnosis includes gallbladder diverticula, gallbladder fold, Phrygian cap, choledochal cyst, pericholecystic fluid, and focal adenomyomatosis. Simultaneous removal of both gallbladders during surgery is advised to prevent cholecystitis and biliary colic in the remaining organ [27].

7.3 Ectopic gallbladder

An ectopic gallbladder is a rare anatomical anomaly of the biliary system. The biliary system as a whole or just the gallbladder is located in an abnormal anatomical position. Several anatomic locations have been reported in literature. The majority of them can be pathogenic because of related factors such as torsion of the gallbladder, cholestasis, and internal hernia (*via* the foramen of Winslow). Ectopic gallbladder should ideally be diagnosed preoperatively to avoid intra- and post-operative complications and to ensure safe management of the patient's associated conditions [28].

The ectopic gallbladder has an incidence of 0.1–0.7%. It can be found in various positions, including left-sided, transverse, retroperitoneal, or floating. Ectopic gallbladders have also been reported in areas such as the lesser omentum, retroduodenal space, falciform ligament, abdominal wall muscles, and even within the thorax [29].

7.3.1 Left-sided gallbladder

A true left-sided gallbladder is an extremely rare anomaly where the gallbladder lies in the left abdomen without a right-sided round ligament. In contrast, a false left-sided gallbladder is not an abnormality of the gallbladder itself, but rather an issue with the round ligament.

Embryologically, a left-sided gallbladder could happen in two ways: (i) the gallbladder primordium deriving from the normal gallbladder bud (from the hepatic diverticulum) moves to the left side instead of remaining on the right side. In this case, the developing peritoneum forces the gallbladder primordium to stay fixed to the undersurface of the left lobe of the liver. Furthermore, the cystic duct's entry remains normal (with the common bile duct). (ii) There is Vesica fellea duplex or double gallbladder formation, but the right one becomes atrophic and finally disappears, and the left one remains as the main one. In this second case, the cystic duct's entry is abnormal (with the common bile duct or the left hepatic but from the left) [30].

7.3.2 Suprahepatic gallbladder

This variant is the rarest, with an incidence ranging from 0.026% to 0.7%. It is typically associated with a right liver love, which is defective in size. The latter may result from a congenital cause that can lead to cirrhotic hypoplasia, malformation, vascular injury of the liver, or the presence of diffuse cholangiocarcinoma. It is hypothesized that when the right lobe is absent, the gallbladder is reoriented, and the colon is displaced upward. This aligns with reports of suprahepatic gallbladders and the upward migration of the hepatic flexure [31].

8. Microscopic anatomy of the gallbladder

The histology of the gallbladder is similar to most of the intraperitoneal organs and its wall is composed of three layers from the inside out: the mucosa, the muscularis propria and the serosa. The muscularis mucosae and the submucosa are absent in gallbladder.

The mucosa consists of one layer of columnar epithelium with microvilli above the lamina propria. The latter contains mainly vascular and lymphatic tissue together with connective tissue. During the fasting period, when the gallbladder is distended and full of bile, the mucosa is smooth, but when it is not distended (postprandial) a presence of mucosal folds is noted. Even though these folds are irregular and not standard in size, they look similar to the villi of the mucosa of the small bowel. Sometimes In cross-section, there are formations seen in the mucosal folds shown as crypts and looking like tubular glands. However, the true glands are evident only at the neck of the gallbladder.

The muscularis propria contains mainly smooth muscle fibers with tissue made of collagen, nerves, vessels, lymphatics, and fat between them. This layer plays a key role in the expulsion of bile [24].

Starting from the mucosa layer and extending to the layer around the smooth muscles without crossing them, there are crypts that are called Rokitansky-Aschoff sinuses. These are invaginations of the epithelium that look like diverticula and vary in depth and size. Rokitansky-Aschoff sinuses are pathognomonic of chronic cholecystitis but can be found also in the normal gallbladder [32].

The outer layer is the serosa which is present at the area of the gallbladder wall which is not attached to the liver surface. This layer is the visceral peritoneum [24].

9. Frequently used surgical terms based on anatomical landmarks

9.1 The Calot's triangle

It was first described in 1891 by Jean François Calot in his doctoral thesis with the title "De la cholecystectomie." He described it as the isosceles triangle with specific boundaries: inferiorly by the cystic duct, medially by the common hepatic duct, and superiorly by the cystic artery [33].

In the modern era of laparoscopic biliary surgery, a different definition was agreed upon for Calot's triangle, which is the triangle with boundaries superior to the inferior surface of the liver, inferior to the cystic duct, and medial to the common bile duct [32–35]. Another name for the Calot's triangle is the cystohepatic or hepatocystic triangle [33].

9.2 The critical view of safety

This term refers to a specific identification of the anatomical structures of the hepatocystic triangle, which in most cases ensures a safe dissection during cholecystectomy. According to Strasberg et al. [36], the critical view of safety consists of the following elements: (i) identification of two tubular structures leading to the gallbladder after careful dissection of the fibrous tissue of the hepatocystic triangle and (ii) adequate dissection of the gallbladder (one third) from the cystic plate [35]. This is applicable to laparoscopic cholecystectomy, which followed the initial "critical view of safety" of open cholecystectomy in early 1995 [37].

10. Conclusion

A detailed knowledge of the anatomy of the gallbladder plays an essential role in many aspects of clinical practice. From basic surgical assessment in primary care, teaching in medical schools, preoperative management, through to complex surgical procedures and postoperative care, it is essential to have and be aware of all anatomical variations.

Not recognizing these vascular subtleties may result in significant complications such as inadvertent injury to major vessels, persistent bleeding post-operatively, or liver ischemia.

Failure to recognize anatomical subtleties can lead to significant complications such as inadvertent injury to major vessels, persistent postoperative bleeding, liver ischemia, or damage to the bile ducts or other vital structures.

With the availability of modern imaging techniques such as CT angiography or MR angiography, along with intraoperative adjuncts including cholangiography or ICG fluorescence, the surgeon is in a better position to recognize and avoid such perils. As the detailed knowledge regarding nuances of gallbladder anatomy continues to evolve, comprehensive preoperative planning and accurate intraoperative navigation will provide the basis for optimal patient management.

Acknowledgements

The methodology used for this chapter involved searching relevant international literature, including published manuscripts and scientifically proven web-based information, as well as published books.

All authors contributed to collecting data and information from the above sources. After analyzing the data and enriching it with information from their areas of medical expertise, they wrote a draft. They also agreed to review the chapter before submission.

Ioannis Gerogiannis conceived and designed the original idea for this chapter. He revised and approved the final version prior to publication. He also designed all the figures using a drawing display. His signature on each figure confirms its originality and ownership.

Conflict of interest

The authors declare no conflict of interest.

Notes/thanks/other declarations

Figures are designed by Ioannis Gerogiannis using the XP pen Artist Pro 19 (Gen 2) ® Drawing Display with an X3 Pro Slim Stylus.

Author details

Ioannis N. Gerogiannis[1*], Razhan K. Ali[1], Mark Sidhom[1], Georgios Bointas[1] and Eirini Tsoutsou[2]

1 Department of General Surgery, Kingston Hospital, London, UK

2 Department of Thalassaemia, Gennimatas General Hospital, Athens, Greece

*Address all correspondence to: drgerogiannis@gmail.com

References

[1] Oxford English Dictionary. Gall bladder [Internet]. 2025. Available from: https://www.oed.com/dictionary/gall-bladder_n [Accessed: April 1, 2025]

[2] Vakili K, Pomfret EA. Biliary anatomy and embryology. The Surgical Clinics of North America. 2008;**88**(6):1159-1vii. DOI: 10.1016/j.suc.2008.07.001

[3] M'connell RJ. The topographical and applied anatomy of the gall-bladder and bile-ducts. Journal of Anatomy and Physiology. 1915;**49**(Pt 3):286-304

[4] Standring S. Gray's Anatomy: The Anatomical Basis of Clinical Practice. 42th ed. New York: Elsevier; 2020. pp. 1217-1218. ISBN 978-0-7020-7707-4

[5] Dasgupta D, Stringer MD. Cystic duct and Heister's "valves". Clinical Anatomy (New York, N.Y.). 2005;**18**(2):81-87. DOI: 10.1002/ca.20118

[6] Jones MW, Hannoodee S, Young M. Anatomy, abdomen and pelvis: Gallbladder. In: StatPearls [Internet]. Treasure Island (FL): StatPearls Publishing; 2025. [Updated 2022 Oct 31]. Available from: https://www.ncbi.nlm.nih.gov/books/NBK459288/

[7] Sangameswaran K. Variations of cystic duct and its clinical significance. International Journal of Anatomy and Research. 2021;**9**(4):8120-8126. DOI: 10.16965/ijar.2021.167

[8] Wineski LE. Snell's Clinical Anatomy by Regions. 11th ed. Philadelphia: Lippincott Williams & Wilkins; 4 Mar 2024. Available from: https://blackwells.co.uk/bookshop/product/Snells-Clinical-Anatomy-by-Regions-by-Lawrence-E-Wineski-Richard-S-Snell/9781975194093 [Accessed: Jun 15, 2025]

[9] Netter FH. Netter Atlas of Human Anatomy: Classic Regional Approach. 8th ed. Philadelphia: Elsevier; 2022. pp. 284-287

[10] Gupta R, Kumar A, Hariprasad CP, Kumar M. Anatomical variations of cystic artery, cystic duct, and gall bladder and their associated intraoperative and postoperative complications: An observational study. Annals of Medicine and Surgery. 2023;**85**(8):3880-3886. Available from: https://journals.lww.com/annals-of-medicine-and-surgery/fulltext/2023/08000/anatomical_variations_of_cystic_artery,_cystic.18.aspx

[11] Hassan AU, Zargar SA, Malik A, Shah P. Surgical significance of variations in anatomy in the biliary region. International Journal of Research in Medical Sciences. 2013;**1**(3):183-187. DOI: 10.5455/2320-6012.ijrms20130812H

[12] Andall RG, Matusz P, du Plessis M, Ward R, Tubbs RS, Loukas M. The clinical anatomy of cystic artery variations: A review of over 9800 cases. Surgical and Radiologic Anatomy. 2016;**38**(5):529-539. Available from: https://link.springer.com/article/10.1007/s00276-015-1600-y

[13] Chen WJ et al. Analysis of the arterial supply of the extrahepatic bile ducts and its clinical significance. Clinical Anatomy. 1999;**12**(4):245-249. Available from: https://onlinelibrary.wiley.com/doi/10.1002/(SICI)1098-2353(1999)12:4%3C245::AID-CA2%3E3.0.CO;2-W

[14] Ayalew AB. Anatomical variations and clinical relevance of cystic artery: A brief review. European Journal of Anatomy. 2020;**24**(1):69-74. Available from: http://www.eurjanat.com/data/pdf/eja.190415ab.pdf

[15] Saidi H, Karanja TM, Ogengo JA. Variant anatomy of the cystic artery in adult Kenyans. Clinical Anatomy. 2007;**20**(8):943-945. Available from: https://onlinelibrary.wiley.com/doi/full/10.1002/ca.20550

[16] Shetty P, Satheesha NB, Sirasanagandla S. Variant origin of a common trunk of the accessory hepatic artery and cystic artery from the superior mesenteric artery. OA Case Reports. 2013;**2**(7):64. DOI: 10.13172/2052-0077-2-7-726

[17] Mlakar B, Gadžijev EM, Ravnik D, Hribernik M. Anatomical variations of the cystic artery. European Journal of Morphology. 2003;**41**(1):31-34

[18] Prasoon P, Katada T, Miura K, Hirose Y, Sakata J, Wakai T, et al. Cystic artery variations and associated vascular complications in laparoscopic cholecystectomy. In: Digestive System—Recent Advances. London, UK: IntechOpen. Available from: https://www.intechopen.com/chapters/63779; 2018 [Accessed: February 9, 2025]

[19] Kavitha Kamath B. An anatomical study of Moynihan's hump of right hepatic artery and its surgical importance. Journal of the Anatomical Society of India. 2016;**65**:S65-S67

[20] Polguj M, Podgórski M, Hogendorf P, Topol M. Variations of the hepatobiliary vasculature including coexistence of accessory right hepatic artery with unusually arising double cystic arteries: Case report and literature review. Anatomical Science International. 2014;**89**(3):195-198. Available from: https://link.springer.com/article/10.1007/s12565-013-0219-5

[21] Dandekar U, Dandekar K. Cystic artery: Morphological study and surgical significance. Anatomy Research International. 2016;**2016**:1-6

[22] Yi SQ, Ohta T, Tsuchida A, Terayama H, Naito M, Li J, et al. Surgical anatomy of innervation of the gallbladder in humans and *Suncus murinus* with special reference to morphological understanding of gallstone formation after gastrectomy. World Journal of Gastroenterology. 2007;**13**(14):2066-2071. DOI: 10.3748/wjg.v13.i14.2066

[23] van Eijck FC, van Veen RN, Kleinrensink GJ, Lange JF. Hartmann's gallbladder pouch revisited 60 years later. Surgical Endoscopy. 2007;**21**(7):1122-1125. DOI: 10.1007/s00464-006-9058-y

[24] Nasar A, Siddiqui SW, Gupta P, Khan AA, Arora NK. Histological changes of gall bladder mucosa and its correlation with various types of cholelithiasis. Journal of Research in Medical and Dental Science. 2021;**9**(7):211-218

[25] Cañizares Díaz JI, Arrobas Velilla T. La agenesia de la vesícula biliar: Reporte de un caso. Gastroenterología y Hepatología. 2013;**37**:24-27. DOI: 10.1016/j.gastrohep.2013.07.009

[26] Kosmidis CS, Koimtzis GD, Kosmidou MS, Ieridou F, Koletsa T, Zarampouka KT, et al. Gallbladder hypoplasia, a congenital abnormality of the gallbladder: A case report. American Journal of Case Reports. 2017;**18**:1320-1324. DOI: 10.12659/ajcr.905963

[27] Pillay Y. Gallbladder duplication. International Journal of Surgery Case Reports. 2015;**11**:18-20. DOI: 10.1016/j.ijscr.2015.04.002

[28] Al-Tarakji M, AlFkey R, Aljohary H, Sameer M, Muhammad Ali S. Successful surgical management of

unusual gallbladder anatomy through laparoscopic cholecystectomy of ectopic gallbladder. Cureus. 2021;**13**(11):e19884. DOI: 10.7759/cureus.19884

[29] Popli MB, Popli V, Solanki Y. Ectopic gall bladder: A rare case. Saudi Journal of Gastroenterology. 2010;**16**(1):50. DOI: 10.4103/1319-3767.58771

[30] Ishii H, Noguchi A, Onishi M, Takao K, Maruyama T, Taiyoh H, et al. True left-sided gallbladder with variations of bile duct and cholecystic vein. World Journal of Gastroenterology. 2015;**21**(21):6754-6758. DOI: 10.3748/wjg.v21.i21.6754

[31] Hessey JA, Halpin L, Simo KA. Suprahepatic gallbladder. Journal of Gastrointestinal Surgery. 2015;**19**(7):1382-1384. DOI: 10.1007/s11605-015-2771-x

[32] Campos A, Abu, Kamesh M, Hacking C, et al. Gallbladder. Radiopaedia.org; [Internet]. 2024 Available from: https://radiopaedia.org/articles/gallbladder?lang=us [Accessed: Feb 23, 2025]

[33] Abdalla S, Pierre S, Ellis H. Calot's triangle. Clinical Anatomy. 2013;**26**(4):493-501. DOI: 10.1002/ca.22170

[34] Haubrich WS. Calot of the triangle of Calot. Gastroenterology. 2002;**123**:1440

[35] Nagral S. Anatomy relevant to cholecystectomy. Journal of Minimal Access Surgery. 2005;**1**:53-58

[36] Strasberg SM, Brunt LM. Rationale and use of the critical view of safety in laparoscopic cholecystectomy. Journal of the American College of Surgeons. 2010;**211**(1):132-138. DOI: 10.1016/j.jamcollsurg.2010.02.053

[37] Strasberg SM, Hertl M, Soper NJ. An analysis of the problem of biliary injury during laparoscopic cholecystectomy. Journal of the American College of Surgeons. 1995;**180**(1):101-125

Chapter 2

Asymptomatic Cholecystitis: The Versatility of a Simple Clinical Question

Sergey Yurievich Muraviev and Mehrshad Ebrahimnezhad

Abstract

There is uncertainty in the surgical tactics for asymptomatic cholecystitis due to the lack of a unified understanding and variability of the causes affecting differential diagnostics when setting indications for cholecystectomy, leading to errors and the development of postcholecystectomy syndrome. We examined 252 patients with asymptomatic cholecystitis. Single stones were present in 36.9%, and multiple stones – in 45.6%. In 19.8%, there are difficulties with ultrasound visualization, which is why there are errors in identifying signs of chronic inflammation in the gallbladder. Thickened walls of the gallbladder were observed in 72.4% with diseases of the stomach. In 70.5% with the papilla of Vater, considering the presence of this pathology, lipids changed. When assessing pancreatic elastase, moderate pancreatic insufficiency was detected in 47.6% and severe insufficiency in 9.1%. The pancreas was heterogeneous in 64.3% and had calcifications in 18.3% and ductal calcifications in 7.5%. Dilation of the common bile duct by more than 6 mm was observed in 27%, and signs of choledocholithiasis were observed in 16.7%. This led to the fact that in 25% of cases, postcholecystectomy syndrome developed. It is necessary to understand the terminology of asymptomatic cholecystitis and conduct coordinated studies to reduce the frequency of unnecessary cholecystectomies and complications.

Keywords: asymptomatic cholecystitis, tactical errors, cholecystectomy, postcholecystectomy syndrome, preventive planning tactics

1. Introduction

Today, there is no consensus in hepatobiliary surgery on the treatment of patients with asymptomatic cholecystitis. This is largely due to the lack of a clear definition of asymptomatic cholecystitis, and the other reason is that there are no unambiguous uniform clinical guidelines for solving this problem in the world.

Clinicians practically do not discuss the issue of treating symptomatic cholecystitis, which can sometimes lead to life-threatening consequences. In another case, the treatment of asymptomatic cholecystitis becomes a subject of discussion. Some authors write that it is necessary to carefully approach the examination of such patients. Other surgeons often downplay or ignore the problem of asymptomatic cholecystitis. Therefore, a literature search is difficult due to the small number of studies on this topic. When comparing clinical practice and individual sources, it follows that asymptomatic cholecystitis occurs more often than described in the literature. Based on the analysis of the disease course, it is reasonable to assume that the disease will remain asymptomatic for most of the time throughout life, so it is generally accepted that 80% of cases of cholelithiasis have no symptoms at all. Clinical manifestations develop in 1-4% of patients per year; 20% of patients develop symptoms 20 years after diagnosis [1, 2].

In hepatobiliary surgery today, at the beginning of the twenty-first century, we are faced with a dilemma. At the same time, there are few data on the natural history of asymptomatic cholecystitis, and there are still no randomized controlled trials in the period between observation and intervention. At the same time, gallstones are a common public health problem, especially in developed countries. In Western countries, 10-20% of people have gallstones, and the incidence rate has almost tripled in the last 30 years (due in part to improved diagnosis). Due to the increase in life expectancy, asymptomatic cholecystitis becomes a serious geriatric problem, since after 70 years, it reaches 30% of the population and more [3].

Since there is no tactical solution in the world recommendations, most surgeons try to avoid treating such patients. For surgeons, a successful outcome and a sure mistake are equally close, when using of an ambiguous approach, so they make efforts to avoid this pathology. Many surgeons resort to dynamic observation or refer the patient to a gastroenterologist. Others hastily perform the operation, accepting the high risk of developing postcholecystectomy syndrome. Indeed, 10-40% of patients after cholecystectomy have persistent complaints, sometimes arising after a short asymptomatic period [4].

In this chapter, devoted to asymptomatic cholecystitis, we decided to reveal the existing features of the course of asymptomatic cholecystitis, attempts to find tactical solutions and existing problems in hepatobiliary surgery based on our own clinical material from the analysis of patients with asymptomatic gallstones.

2. Global surgical theory of asymptomatic Cholecystitis: A literature review

2.1 Materials and methods

During the preliminary literature search in high-evidence databases: PubMed/Medline, semanticscholar.org, and scholar.google.com, we used words and phrases: "asymptomatic cholecystitis", "latent cholecystitis", "calculous cholecystitis", "silent gallstones", "asymptomatic gallstones", "cholecystectomy for asymptomatic cholecystitis". All articles retrieved from the search were transferred to the Rayyan platform, which simplified the selection of publications and excluded duplicate studies. Each of the authors, independent of the other, read all abstracts and applied the Oxford Centre inclusion and exclusion criteria. Then, a third independent author did the same process. The selected publications were classified according to the level of evidence from I to V grade and recommendations from A to D according to evidence-based medicine and AGREED II (Appraisal Of Guidelines For Research & Evaluation II). Finally, we applied the preferred reporting items for systematic reviews and meta-analyses (PRISMA) system (e.g., **Figure 1**), which allowed us to methodologically select each study. They were then reviewed in detail to draw the conclusions presented in our review.

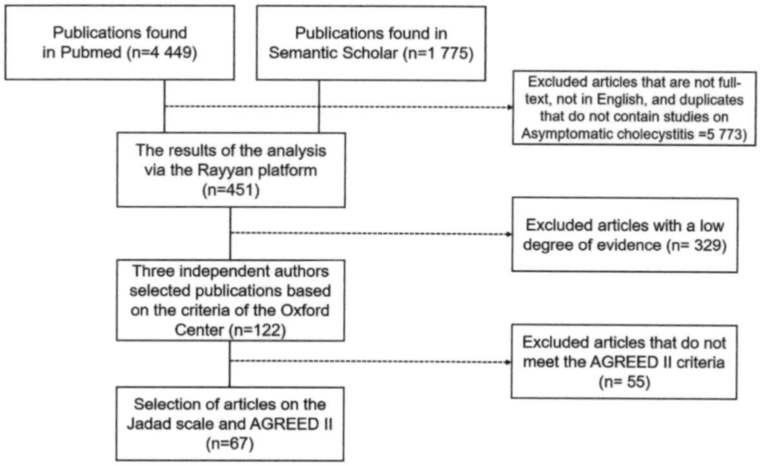

Figure 1.
The block diagram of the analysis of publications according to the PRISMA algorithm.

For mutual understanding between the author and the reader, we consider it necessary to conduct an excursion into the problem of terminology of hepatobiliary surgery associated with asymptomatic cholecystitis. First of all, we emphasize that surgeons still do not have a clear understanding of the term "asymptomatic cholecystitis". Many surgeons and researchers wonder whether there is a substitution of the concepts of "asymptomatic cholecystitis" and "asymptomatic choledocholithiasis". We believe that it is impossible to conduct discussions without a clear clarification of the terminology due to the resulting confusion, confusion, and errors in judgment.

Indeed, there are many recommendations in the literature on asymptomatic choledocholithiasis. They are indicated by several world-class clinical guidelines from national guidelines from the National Institute for Health and Care Excellence in the UK (NICE), the European Society of Gastrointestinal Endoscopy (ESGE), the British Society of Gastroenterology (BSG), and the European Association for the Study of the Liver (EASL) to Tokyo Guide (2018) [5–9]. Focusing primarily on the removal of stones from the common bile duct by different procedures, the conclusion of three of these recommendations (NICE, ESGE, and BSG) indicates that research into the management of patients with asymptomatic cholecystitis is an important priority for the scientific community dealing with cholelithiasis.

The EASL discussion on the treatment of patients with asymptomatic stones includes a weak recommendation based on very low-quality evidence [8]. However, their decision is justified by the risk that in postcholecystectomy patients, preoperative symptoms of unknown etiology may persist or appear periodically.

In the ESGE and EASL guidelines, the term "asymptomatic cholecystitis" is replaced by two different concepts: "asymptomatic cholecystolithiasis", and "silent gallstones", the latter being used more often [10]. In this case, asymptomatic cholelithiasis is defined as the presence of stones in the gallbladder without clinical manifestations (colic, jaundice, pancreatitis). Agreeing with this terminology, the authors of the American College of Gastroenterology (ACG) Guideline on Gallstone Disease (2021) state that stones detected incidentally on ultrasound that do not cause symptoms are called "Silent gallstones" and do not support prophylactic cholecystectomy in such patients [11].

According to information from the medical resource UpToDate, "Approach to the patient with incidental gallstones" (2023), there is a term "asymptomatic gallstones" – this is a condition in which the patient does not have episodes of biliary colic or inflammation. Cholecystectomy in this situation is not recommended unless there are signs of complications (cholecystitis, cholangitis, and pancreatitis) [12].

Thus, the term "silent gallstones" or "asymptomatic cholecystolithiasis" is more often used in the literature, rather than "asymptomatic cholecystitis", since cholecystitis, by definition, implies inflammation (i.e., symptoms). If there is no inflammation, it is more correct to speak of asymptomatic gallstones.

It is also important to note that in ICD-11 (International Classification of Diseases, 11th revision), asymptomatic cholecystitis is classified in section DC11.0 – Cholecystitis without stones (acalculous cholecystitis). If "asymptomatic cholecystitis" means chronic cholecystitis without clinical manifestations (e.g., accidentally detected during an ultrasound or other examination), then another code can be used: DC11.9 – Cholecystitis, unspecified (if there is no specification for the presence of stones), DC11.0 – Acalculous cholecystitis (if the absence of stones is confirmed). If there is cholecystolithiasis (stones in the gallbladder) without symptoms, then this is coded separately: DC11.2 – Gallstones without cholecystitis.

However, the term "asymptomatic cholecystitis" does exist, and it does not reflect a diagnosis, but a pathological process in the gallbladder in the presence of stones, which has its own course, clinical manifestations, and complications that require treatment, both conservative and surgical. Therefore, there is no need to include the term "asymptomatic calculous cholecystitis" separately. At the same time, we adhere to the global concept that asymptomatic acalculous cholecystitis is not a clinical problem and will not be discussed in this chapter.

We agree with surgeons who claim that cholecystitis itself implies inflammation of the gallbladder wall. But at the same time, the destructive process in the gallbladder wall can occur without acute inflammation, and then we can interpret this pathology as "chronic cholecystitis". Undoubtedly, asymptomatic cholecystitis occurs with the development of chronic inflammation and often with the restructuring of the gallbladder wall into fibrosis or fat deposits. "Asymptomatic cholecystitis" has clinical symptoms, but they are hidden behind the clinical manifestations of other organs, and it is almost impossible to isolate them from the complex of symptoms. Therefore, we can say that differential diagnostics requires first removing the "masks" of clinical symptoms of other diseases. The course of "asymptomatic cholecystitis" is due to the slow development of the pathological process, which has no patterns and rules and often manifests itself after an exacerbation of another related pathology. Just like vice versa, after cholecystectomy, several complaints disappear, and only those remain that were not related to gallbladder disease. Complications with "asymptomatic cholecystitis" can also develop, especially the very same symptomatic or asymptomatic choledocholithiasis, which requires surgical treatment, and because of this, there is a world discussion about performing preventive cholecystectomy.

Therefore, further in our chapter, we will talk about asymptomatic cholecystitis as a pathological condition of the gallbladder wall, arising as a result of the lithogenic properties of bile, accompanied by cholesterosis or chronic destruction of the wall, leading to dyskinesia of the gallbladder and biliary tract, accompanied by periodically occurring cholestasis, leading to biliary hypertension due to increased tone of the sphincters of Oddi and the gallbladder, causing an erased clinical picture, similar to a number of diseases of the gastrointestinal tract and hepatobiliary-pancreatoduodenal zone, having a favorable prognosis, but for a number of reasons sometimes complicated by choledocholithiasis, mechanical jaundice, acute cholecystitis or pancreatitis.

The essence of the disease "asymptomatic cholecystitis" is that it is a clinical complex of etiologically based pathogenetically interrelated changes in the organs of the hepatobiliarypancreatoduodenal zone, in contrast to "asymptomatic cholecystolithiasis", "asymptomatic gallstones" or "silent gallstones". Such a condition as "asymptomatic gallstones" or " silent gallstones " does not require active surgical tactics, and performing preventive cholecystectomy seems ephemeral. In this, we fully support the global clinical recommendations. However, asymptomatic cholecystitis with its pathogenic effect on the pancreas and duodenum, and the risks of complications in the form of choledocholithiasis or papillitis of the large duodenal papilla causes concern in a surgeon who understands the essence and depth of this pathophysiological process. And this is the dilemma of surgeons in performing cholecystectomy or refusing it in favor of a wait-and-see tactic of monitoring the course of the disease.

Many people note that the term "asymptomatic cholecystitis" can easily be confused with "asymptomatic choledocholithiasis". However, in their definition, these are completely different processes that can occur interconnectedly, can be a consequence of each other, or can be parallel and independent of each other. Indeed, with asymptomatic cholecystitis, choledocholithiasis without clinical manifestations can occur, but mechanical jaundice can also develop. In our practice, we have encountered asymptomatic cholecystitis and separately occurring choledocholithiasis with obvious clinical manifestations of intermittent jaundice. Therefore, the authors consider any objection regarding the confusion in our understanding of these two pathological processes to be wrong and reserve the right to public discussion in literary form if disagreements arise on this matter.

Thus, today it seems that the global community is avoiding addressing the issue of chronic cholecystitis, narrowing the extensive pathological process and symptom complex to simple gall stone under the terms "asymptomatic cholecystolithiasis," "asymptomatic gallstones " or " silent gallstones " and limited surgical tactics to the development of gallstone complications. In view of this, we provide a literature review of the state and issues of tactics in hepatobiliary surgery for asymptomatic cholecystitis in world practice.

2.2 Views on asymptomatic cholecystitis and approaches to it

In the global surgical community, when considering the course of asymptomatic cholecystitis, there is an opinion that never has a clear clinical picture. All that doctors pay attention to is a combination of two facts: periodic pain in the right hypochondrium and the presence of stones in the gallbladder; the latter are often detected during screening examinations of the abdominal cavity.

Indeed, the issue of asymptomatic cholecystitis and the presence or absence of its specific clinical picture is still controversial. This is largely due to changes in the internal organs occurring simultaneously with the pathology of the gallbladder and having their own clinical symptoms. Such a multitude of symptoms causes confusion in recognizing obvious signs of cholecystitis with asymptomatic stones. Its symptoms are similar to dysfunction and exacerbations of diseases of the internal organs, especially with the progression of cholelithiasis, accompanied by morphological changes in the intestine, pancreas, or stomach.

By analogy with asymptomatic cholecystitis, there are reports that during a 15-year course of asymptomatic choledocholithiasis, its specific clinical signs were confirmed only in 11.5%, and then on average 3.4 years after the detection of stones in the common bile duct. In this case, the main complaints of patients were colic in the right hypochondrium, accompanied by jaundice and fever, associated with the development of cholangitis [13].

The patient's doubts about the necessity of surgical intervention are dispelled by the surgeon's argument about the risk of possible complications associated with long-term presence of stones in the gallbladder. Small stones blocking the sphincter of Oddi can also cause distal obstruction and acute pancreatitis [14]. Thus, there are observations that the course of asymptomatic cholecystitis more often leads to complications than cholecystitis with clinical manifestations (26.4% versus 11.7%, $P < 0.01$) [15]. At the same time, the severity of complications that develop in patients with asymptomatic cholecystitis is significantly higher and more dangerous than in clinically expressed gallbladder pathology (group with asymptomatic cholecystitis – 16.1%, group with symptoms – 3.7%, $R = 0.036$) [16]. However, it is important to clarify that against the background of "apparent well-being", 32% of patients with asymptomatic cholecystitis after endoscopic lithoextraction experienced side effects in the form of exacerbation of symptoms, in 5.2% associated with acute severe pancreatitis [17].

There are few studies on asymptomatic cholecystitis, and there is no uniformity in the available publications. For example, when treating patients for asymptomatic cholecystitis with symptoms or complications caused by common bile duct stones, the best-known national guidelines recommend that stone removal be offered [18]. However, this consensus is not present when discussing cases of occult gallstones that may be detected during cholecystectomy by endoscopic ultrasound examination (EUS) or intraoperative cholangiography (IOC), or detected during abdominal imaging performed for other reasons.

The concept of expectant therapy is also controversial, with a statistically lower cumulative incidence of biliary complications, 6.1% at 1 year, 11% at 3 years, and 17% at 5 years [19]. Although asymptomatic stone clearance was observed in 19% of patients [20]. Cholecystectomy may not be indicated for patients with asymptomatic gallstones and gallbladder polyps measuring 5 mm in diameter [21].

Today, few doctors and scientists are trying to solve the problem of managing patients with asymptomatic cholecystitis before surgery. Surgeons mainly deal with complications or missed pathology after cholecystectomy. This is wrong. Even after a successful cholecystectomy, with a satisfactory result for the surgeon and a good surgical technique and positive outcome, the presence of previous complaints in patients or the appearance of new symptoms causes anxiety, and sometimes panic, and reluctance to deal with such patients. This difficult clinical situation may also be associated with the laparoscopic technique of cholecystectomy, in contrast to those physicians who consider it impeccable. When choosing any operation, patients with asymptomatic cholecystitis should be examined comprehensively to substantiate all complaints and symptoms present in the preoperative period. As an example, an analysis of the literature showed that in recent studies, preoperative dyspepsia was not considered as a factor contributing to the development of postcholecystectomy syndrome. This discovery may contribute to understanding the pathophysiology of postcholecystectomy syndrome [22].

2.3 Differential diagnosis of asymptomatic cholecystitis

To a surgeon starting his journey in hepatobiliary surgery, at first glance, it will seem that the abbreviation "asymptomatic cholecystitis" contains the true meaning of the words: inflammation of the gallbladder that occurs without clinical symptoms. However, this is not the case. In practice, this misconception is quickly cleared up with the correct, thorough, and detailed collection of complaints and the history of the disease, identifying all the symptoms present in a patient assessed as having "asymptomatic cholecystitis". In fact, with a thoughtful approach, many diseases, such as esophagitis, hernia of the esophageal opening of the diaphragm, gastritis, duodenitis, duodenostasis, colitis, ureteral colic, glomerulonephritis, pyelitis, etc., can mask cholecystitis. This is when a patient examined by a doctor with several complaints and an unclear clinical picture receives a diagnosis related to the manifestations of the current leading disease, and at this moment, cholecystitis can be "sort of" asymptomatic. However, the manifestations of asymptomatic cholecystitis are not related to the clinical picture, and its structural changes and dysfunction "secretly" or implicitly lead to organ pathology accompanied by a bright and obvious clinical picture. Such indirect participation of asymptomatic cholecystitis in the pathology of the abdominal organs creates certain "masks" of asymptomatic cholecystitis. The same is true with concomitant kidney pathology or osteochondrosis of the spine with radiculopathy and intercostal neuralgia, which may have clinical symptoms similar to chronic cholecystitis, including asymptomatic ones. After cholecystectomy, when the gallbladder is removed, the patient still has pathology of other organs and complaints and symptoms return again or new ones appear due to disorganization in the absence of the gallbladder. Every experienced surgeon should not forget that under the mask of asymptomatic cholecystitis, which is considered an indication of cholecystectomy or conservative treatment, a completely different pathology may be hidden. We will present the most significant information about this in this subsection.

According to many authors, gallstone disease is a consequence of chronic pancreatitis. Therefore, the clinical picture can proceed in a similar manner and often with more pronounced symptoms of pancreatic pathology. But in this situation, there are many points that require clarification. There is still no clear evidence that asymptomatic calculous cholecystitis is a consequence of chronic pancreatitis. In fact, many surgeons in their clinical practice miss the fact about exocrine pancreatic insufficiency, which occurs in chronic pancreatitis, causing a disturbance in lipid metabolism in the body and ultimately, an increase in lipids in the bile.

At the same time, there is still no convincing evidence of the connection between dyslipidemia and the lithogenic properties of bile. Thus, there are studies showing an inverse relationship between cholesterol and bile acids in the blood and their concentration in bile when biliary stones occur. At the same time, it is difficult to track the level of lipids in the blood over a long period of time, and its point indicators during analysis may not be constant.

But it is very important to clarify another thing, the gallbladder itself has an exocrine function since it secretes such active substances as secretin and cholecystokinin. Secretin is a hormone that stimulates the pancreas, and bile, entering the duodenum, promotes the release of secretin, which enhances the secretion of bicarbonates by the S cells of the pancreas, neutralizing gastric acid and creating an optimal pH for pancreatic enzymes [23]. Cholecystokinin (CCK), secreted in response to fats, stimulates gallbladder contraction and secretion of pancreatic enzymes, participating in the coordination of the gallbladder and pancreas [24]. Thus, the gallbladder indirectly affects the pancreas and gastrointestinal tract through hormonal mechanisms along the CCK-dependent stimulation pathway and bile acids upon activation of FXR/TGR5 and thus, stimulation of secretin [25]. Given this, it is important to understand that with asymptomatic cholecystitis, excretory dysfunction of the gallbladder still occurs.

This affects the activity of the pancreas, which leads to its morphologic restructuring and exocrine insufficiency accompanied by dyslipidemia and clinical manifestations of chronic pancreatitis.

Violation of the qualitative properties of bile, the excretory function of the gallbladder, and violation of coordination in the interaction of the gallbladder and pancreas leads to pathology of the duodenum. Surgeons practicing hepatobiliary surgery need to understand this and take it into account in the differential diagnosis of duodenitis and asymptomatic cholecystitis.

Pathology of the duodenum is the most typical error in the indication for cholecystectomy. Pain in the epigastrium and right hypochondrium is very similar to colic in the gallbladder. But for some reason, surgeons do not consider it valuable to additionally examine all parts of the duodenum in patients with asymptomatic cholecystitis or limit themselves to examining the ampulla and duodenum.

At the same time, inflammation in the duodenum, often associated with dyskinesia of the pyloroduodenal junction and incoordination of the gallbladder and pancreas, and the resulting duodenostasis lead to increased pressure in the lumen of the duodenum. The outflow of bile from the common bile duct occurs mainly under the suction effect of the duodenum or under the influence of intraductal pressure. Cholecystokinin is not released from the I-cells of the duodenum, causing no contraction of the gallbladder and stimulating the secretion of enzymes by the pancreas [26]. The resulting duodenostasis leads to hypertension in the lumen of the duodenum, thereby further blocking the secretion of bile, especially when it thickens. Bile secretion is impaired, and this is what causes the clinical picture of sudden pain in the right hypochondrium. In view of this, it is wrong to assess the condition of the duodenum as a diagnosis with treatment tactics without taking into account asymptomatic cholecystitis. This is what causes the progression of the disease due to incorrectly chosen diagnostic tactics and errors in treatment.

Thus, in one study, 200 patients were examined after cholecystectomy with persistent complaints of the same pain in the right hypochondrium [27]. Moreover, in 10.2% of cases, microcrystals were detected during microscopy of duodenal bile. The authors noted that with the use of ursodeoxycholic acid for several months, complaints of pain significantly decreased or disappeared [28]. These data confirmed that the cause of the pain was microlithiasis accompanying the course of asymptomatic cholecystitis, and cholecystectomy was not justified in all cases. In such cases, preoperative tactics in patients with any cholecystitis should include a set of diagnostic methods, including supplemented by the detection and confirmation of microlithiasis. Thus, the use of microscopy of duodenal or hepatic bile obtained during duodenal intubation could determine its truly asymptomatic course in patients with cholecystitis and exclude surgical intervention [29].

At the same time, given the asymptomatic course of cholecystitis, many nonspecific symptoms of gallstones in cholelithiasis can be identified with possible underlying diseases, such as duodenogastroesophageal reflux and sphincter of Oddi dysfunction, functional dyspepsia, irritable bowel syndrome, which often seem to be more likely causes of complaints [30–34].

It is generally accepted that bile affects the condition of the colon. Indeed, bile acids modulate the composition of the intestinal microflora, which in turn affects the health of the gastrointestinal tract, inflammation, and even the function of the pancreas along the intestine-pancreas axis [35]. When colitis occurs during the recirculation of substances through the portal vein system through bile, a chronic inflammatory environment arises both in the intestine and in the biliary system. There are studies confirming the fact that biliary tract diseases depend on the microbiota of the colon, for example, biliary cholangitis, primary sclerosing cholangitis, and even cirrhosis of the liver [36]. In this can a situation is possible without the development of a biliary tract infection but causing and maintaining subacute inflammation in the gallbladder itself. Chronic inflammatory response in the intestines and gallbladder alters the function of the reticuloendothelial system and affects the biochemical composition of bile.

There are currently few studies on patients with asymptomatic gallstones associated with changes in gut microbiota, and they do not take into account the influence of metabolic factors on gut microbiota. One study found that in asymptomatic cholecystitis, the diversity and abundance of gut microbiota were significantly reduced compared to healthy individuals [37]. It is known that changes in the composition of the intestinal flora are associated with the metabolic syndrome accompanying obesity, diabetes, and hypertension, all of which occur with high frequency in gallstones, indicating a connection between gallstones and dysbiosis [38]. This is confirmed in another study, which showed that gut microbiota changes at different levels of the intestine in the presence of gallstones [39].

Therefore, it is impossible to deny the role of asymptomatic cholecystitis in the development of acute and chronic colitis with dysbacteriosis phenomena and the entire clinical picture of these diseases. It is possible to deny the fact of participation of asymptomatic cholecystitis in the clinic of colitis, but it is impossible not to take into account that the altered gallbladder itself as a separate pathogenetic link affects the choice of treatment tactics in gastroenterology and hepatobiliary surgery.

Renal dysmorphism due to glomerulonephritis or pyelonephritis is another pathology that can lead to errors in the management of patients with asymptomatic cholecystitis, and it must be conspired. It also perplexes physicians when a patient with asymptomatic cholecystitis has urolithiasis, especially with signs of ureteral colic [40]. Apparently, this issue remains in the shadow of the views of the surgical community. This issue is rarely raised in discussions but remains relevant for most surgeons today. Patients with a history of gallstones have an increased risk of developing nephrolithiasis, and residual or recurrent biliary disease after cholecystectomy may contribute to the development of kidney-related symptoms [41]. There is some evidence that renal pathology may be a cause of postcholecystectomy syndrome. In some cases, undiagnosed renal colic or ureteral obstruction may be misinterpreted as postcholecystectomy pain in a patient with asymptomatic cholecystitis, highlighting the need for urologic evaluation [42]. Sometimes in asymptomatic cholecystitis, renal dysfunction, especially nephrolithiasis or ureteral obstruction, may mimic stone migration, as a variant of Mirizzi syndrome, and cause symptoms including chronic abdominal pain and dyspepsia [43].

2.4 The course of asymptomatic cholecystitis

In the modern clinical practice of hepatobiliary surgeons, therapists, and gastroenterologists, asymptomatic cholecystitis is a very common pathology. This is due to two main reasons: improving the quality of hardware diagnostics and digitalization of data recording. The introduction of a new approach to examination standards with the widespread use of ultrasound examination of the abdominal cavity, including with unclear abdominal pain, and clinical observation of patients with asymptomatic cholecystitis made it possible to identify a benign course of the disease. Overall, over a long-term follow-up of 6.9 years on average, 1-4% of patients with asymptomatic cholecystitis develop any associated symptoms or complications annually from the time of diagnosis [44]. Asymptomatic cholecystitis develops into symptomatic gallstone disease in 10% of patients within 5 years and in 20% by the age of 20 [45]. Moreover, even if a patient with asymptomatic cholecystitis experiences a single symptomatic episode similar to gallstone disease, the probability that it will not recur is only 58.5% in mild cases and 52.1% in cases of moderate severity [46]. It is also important to note that with careful attention to collecting complaints and medical history before the occurrence of any complication associated with asymptomatic cholecystitis, it is almost always preceded by pain identical to acute cholecystitis, cholangitis, and acute pancreatitis, regardless of the duration of the disease [2]. Therefore, it is important to consider that aging may be associated with a higher risk of developing symptoms [16].

Another finding in asymptomatic cholecystitis is the possible calcification of the gallbladder known as porcelain gallbladder (PGB). The term PGB originally referred to the blue discoloration and brittle consistency of the gallbladder wall, but it is often used to describe all types of gallbladder calcification. When extensive calcium deposits invade the gallbladder, the gallbladder wall may become brittle and blue, resulting in a porcelain appearance. Other names for this condition are calcific gallbladder or calcific cholecystitis [47]. Porcelain gallbladder is an extremely rare condition with an incidence of 0.06 to 0.8% and is associated with cholelithiasis in 90% of cases [48]. Porcelain gallbladder was originally considered a premalignant condition, although it has become more commonly considered benign, with autopsy reports of an incidence of porcelain gallbladder as high as 1.1% [49].

Patients with porcelain gallbladder often complain of biliary tract pain or even a palpable hard mass in the right upper quadrant [47]. However, the diagnosis is often made when calcification is detected as an incidental finding on routine abdominal x-ray, sonography, and computed tomography scans done for some other reason. CT is considered the investigation of choice because it can accurately differentiate it from other pathologies. In addition, there are several conditions that can closely mimic porcelain gallbladder, such as large opaque gallstones, calcified liver hydatid cysts, metastatic deposits, calcified renal cysts, schistosomiasis, calcified lymph nodes, and other granulomatous diseases [48].

Data on the asymptomatic course of porcelain cyst are scattered, which may be associated with the interpretation of the histological picture. Thus, according to some data, out of 1608 cases of patients with cholecystectomy, 13 (0.81%) had a porcelain cyst, of which 4 (31%) were asymptomatic, according to others, out of 113 patients, 79 (70%) were asymptomatic [50, 51].

Another problem is the presence of biliary sludge. There is little information in the literature on the study of this process, and the published data have a low level of evidence and recommendations. However, in the case of patients with asymptomatic cholecystitis, cholestasis with biliary sludge has preoperative risks of surgical complications. In view of this, indirectly suspected biliary sludge requires verification, and if detected, treatment may be similar to microlithiasis of the biliary tract [52].

The combination of asymptomatic cholecystitis with incidentally detected asymptomatic choledocholithiasis is one of the controversial issues in the management of such patients. This situation is accompanied by a number of tactical decisions related to possible complications of choledocholithiasis and the indication for prophylactic cholecystectomy [53].

Today, despite the recommendations, there are supporters of active cholecystectomy for any pain syndrome in the right hypochondrium similar to the symptoms of typical biliary colic, sometimes exaggerating any abdominal symptoms while some surgeons consider asymptomatic cholecystitis as a benign disease, complications of which are rare. Unfortunately, the recommendations do not provide a clear scheme for the management of such patients, although they suggest a thorough examination, they do not contain any definitive methods of treating the patient, and the resulting unregulated approach to the management of asymptomatic cholecystitis leads to ongoing debates between scientific communities, and patients suffer.

There are many reports that patients who have undergone cholecystectomy suffer from persistent pain or other abdominal symptoms, with asymptomatic cholecystitis reaching 40% [54]. Therefore, the course of asymptomatic cholecystitis should be considered in conjunction with the typical picture of pain in the biliary tract or with what has developed with a certain complication of gallstone disease (choledocholithiasis, cholangitis, cholecystitis, and pancreatitis).

Mortality due to asymptomatic gallstones is extremely rare, accounting for 3-7% of all cholelithiasis-related deaths, usually in the elderly, due to biliary or postoperative complications [55]. Autopsies show that more than 90% of patients with cholelithiasis die from causes unrelated to the disease [46].

2.5 Issues of treatment tactics for patients with asymptomatic cholecystitis

All existing clinical guidelines consider the treatment tactics for patients with asymptomatic cholecystitis only from two sides: firstly, whether to perform a cholecystectomy or not, and secondly, whether there is concomitant choledocholithiasis or not, and if so, to perform planned treatment in a surgical hospital. The Russian guidelines for cholecystitis for 2024 consider the treatment of specifically "asymptomatic cholecystolithiasis", and not "asymptomatic cholecystitis" [56]. At the same time, the issue of other conditions concomitant with asymptomatic cholecystitis, such as pathology of the pancreas, stomach, duodenum, and colon, is not addressed. Also, today's guidelines do not have a clear scheme for managing patients with asymptomatic cholecystitis. A thorough examination is assumed, but there is no indication for what tactical purpose it is necessary to carry it out in this volume, so any connection with determining the final method of treatment of the patient is lost, which leads to an ongoing debate among scientific circles and puts surgeons in a dilemma.

The EASL guidelines do not recommend treating patients with asymptomatic cholecystitis, which is a weak recommendation because symptoms may persist even after cholecystectomy [8]. The Russian cholecystitis guidelines for 2024 and three national guidelines (NICE, ESGE and BSG) support surgery only for asymptomatic choledocholithiasis, but not for asymptomatic cholecystitis, leaving surgeons with a dilemma whether to perform surgery or not [5–7, 56].

However, conservative treatment with clinical supervision is recognized throughout the world as possible and safe, while even with laparoscopic cholecystectomy there is a mortality rate, albeit low (<0.2%) [57]. While a number of studies show the cost-effectiveness of the laparoscopic method taking into account the clinical course of asymptomatic or minimally symptomatic gallstones, observation of a patient with asymptomatic cholecystitis is a cheaper option than performing any surgical intervention, including prophylactic cholecystectomy [58]. Also, the benefits of cholecystectomy for the prevention of complications remain unproven, and a selective approach may be justified to avoid unnecessary risks and costs. Furthermore, although laparoscopic cholecystectomy is considered a safe procedure with a mortality rate of less than 0.2% and a complication rate of less than 5.0%, in patients with asymptomatic cholecystitis, surgery, and general anesthesia are considered risky compared to conservative treatment or observation [17, 58]. Unfortunately, cholecystectomy cannot guarantee the resolution of clinical manifestations identified during preoperative examination.

The benefits of routine prophylactic cholecystectomy remain unproven, and a selective approach may be justified to avoid unnecessary risks and costs. Indications for preventive cholecystectomy may be given to those patients with asymptomatic cholecystitis who present with ischemic heart disease due to the increased likelihood of complications with acute cholecystitis after 5 years of follow-up [59]. Another indication for cholecystectomy is pregnancy planning, as the risk of complications is significantly increased, and the consequences may be fatal for the fetus. However, in asymptomatic gallstone disease during pregnancy, it is indicated that no special treatment measures are required; the use of ursodeoxycholic acid (UDCA) preparations for the prevention of gallstone formation or dissolution during pregnancy is contraindicated [56]. However, taking ursodeoxycholic acid to dissolve gallstones is not effective, although dissolution of stones was observed in 2.2% of patients who did not take ursodeoxycholic acid [60].

At the same time, a significant disadvantage of the long-term course of asymptomatic cholecystitis and the management of such patients by conservative methods is that gallstone disease does not proceed without consequences. In any case, they develop asymptomatic pathology of other organs, for example, chronic pancreatitis, duodenitis, and if these patients have chronic liver diseases, including cirrhosis of the liver, the frequency of complications and mortality associated with cholecystectomy is higher compared to patients without them.

3. An integrated approach to assessing the condition of a patient with asymptomatic cholecystitis

We examined 252 patients with asymptomatic cholecystitis (e.g., **Table 1**). Ultrasound data indicated that the size of the gallbladder did not have any significant changes characteristic of gallstone, accompanied by chronic inflammation of the organ.

All parameters of the gallbladder according to the ultrasound scan were at an average level: length – 66.85 ± 1.038 mm, width – 28.63 ± 0.371 mm. The ratio of the length/width of the gallbladder was equal to 2.7. The gallbladder volume in asymptomatic cholecystitis on average was 26.72 ± 0.975 ml, and the area was 14.62 ± 1.384 cm^2. The thickness of the gallbladder wall was 2.67 ± 0.392 mm; a single polyp was detected on its surface at 6.7%.

It is important to note that a third of the population, or 36.9% of patients, had gallbladder deformation. The most common form was pear-shaped at 40.1%. Oval and oblong forms were in 12.3% and 10.7% of cases, respectively.

Cholesterosis was present in 18.7% of gallbladders, of which the focal reticulate form was found in 4.3%, the diffuse reticulate form in 7.9%, the mixed reticulate-polyposis form in 4.8%, and the polyposis form in 1.6%. Thus, the conclusion suggests that cholesterosis of the gallbladder reflects only the direct morphofunctional state of the gallbladder and not the clinical picture of asymptomatic cholecystitis. Therefore, cholesterosis itself cannot be an indication of cholecystectomy.

In asymptomatic cholecystitis, in 36.9% of cases, there were single stones in the gallbladder, and multiple in 45.6%. Analyzing the importance of gallbladder contents

Index	Value	Index	Value
Men/women	56/22.2%/196/77.8%	Gallbladder index	
Age	46.85 ± 1.295	Gallbladder length, mm	66.85 ± 1.038
Triglycerides, mmol/l	1.16 ± 0.834	Gallbladder width, mm	28.63 ± 0.371
HDL-C, mmol/l	1.23 ± 0.737	Gallbladder form	
Total cholesterol, mmol/l	5.19 ± 1.237	Pear-shaped Gallbladder	101/40.1%
Glucose, mmol/l	4.67 ± 0.848	Oval	31/12.3%
Insulin,	5.64 ± 1.195	Oblong	27/10.7%
Waist circumference, cm	81.01 ± 1.385	Deformation	93/36.9%
BMI, kg/m2	24.45 ± 1.846	Gallbladder volume, ml	26.72 ± 0.975
LAP, cm x mmol/l	16.91 ± 0.269	Gallbladder area, sq. ^{2}	14.62 ± 1.384
Atherogenic Index (AI)	3.61 ± 0.281	Length to width ratio A/B	2.7
Atherogenic index of plasma (AIP)	−0.27 ± 0.013	Gallbladder wall thickness, mm	2.67 ± 0.392
Homeostatic Model Assessment of Insulin Resistance (HOMA-IR)	1.63 ± 0.897	Single polyp of the gallbladder	17/6.7%
Ultrasound signs of liver steatosis		Cholesterosis of the gallbladder	47/18.7%
Without liver pathology	51/20.2%	Focal reticular form	11 / 4.3%
Hepatomegaly	54/21.4%	Diffuse mesh form	20 /7, 9%
Diffuse hyperechogenicity of the liver ("bright liver")	76/30.2%	Mixed reticulate-polypous form	1 2 / 4, 8%
Increased echogenicity of the liver compared to the kidneys	71/28.2%	Polypous form	4/1.6%
Vascular pattern blurring	81/32.1%	Low-echo positive suspension ("sludge")	44/17.4%
Distal echo attenuation	65/25.8%	Single stones	93/36.9%
NLFS	0.39 ± 0.026	Multiple stones	115/45.6%
DBPTRI	3.81 ± 0.375	Pancreas index	
FLI	54.7 ± 2.702	head	3.8 2 ± 1.523
Characteristics of the biliary tract		body	2.94 ± 0.642
Without pathology of the biliary tract	97/38.5%	tail	2.97 ± 1.467
dilation of the common bile duct (> 6 мм)	68/27%	The contours are uneven	163/64.7%
stones within the common bile ducts	42/16.7%	The contours are even	89/35.3%
Bile duct cysts	21/8.3%	The density is hyperechoic	151/59.9%
Dysfunction of the biliary tract		The density is isoechoic	72/28.6%
Normokinesis	38/15.1%	The density is hypoechoic	29/11.5%
Hyperkinesis	50/19.8%	The structure is homogeneous	90/35.7%

Index	Value	Index	Value
Hypokinesis	164/65.1%	The structure is heterogeneous oh	162/64.3%
Associated pathology		Pancreatic calcifications:	
Gastroesophageal reflux disease	29/11.5%	Parenchyma	46/18.3%
Superficial gastritis	34/13.5%	Ductal	19/7.5%
Erosive gastritis	4/1.6%	Pancreatic duct:	
Gastric ulcer	9/3.6%	dilation of the lateral ducts >2 мм	44/17.5%
Duodenogastric reflux	28/11.1%	Wirsung duct (ductus pancreaticus) > 5 мм	24/9.5%
Erosive duodenitis	6/2.4%	Pseudocysts of the pancreas	11/4.4%
Ulcer of the duodenum	3/1.2%	Exocrine insufficiency	
Diverticula of the duodenum	2/0.8%	Function saved	17/6.7%
Stenosis of the ampulla of Vater	18/7. %	Easy	92/36.5%
Hypertonicity of the sphincter of Oddi	16/6.3%	Moderate	120/47.6%
Hypotonicity of the sphincter of Oddi	10/4%	Heavy	23/9.1%

Table 1.
Characteristics of patients with asymptomatic cholecystitis.

for choosing surgical treatment tactics, we found that in 17.4% of cases, the gallbladder contained low-echo positive suspension ("sludge").

Thus, the ultrasound picture of the gallbladder indicated a situation in which patients with a small, deformed gallbladder filled with multiple stones were more often subjected to surgical intervention. For this reason, postcholecystectomy syndrome most often develops in them. Patients with medium sized gallbladders with single polyps or stones, as well as with cholesterol or "sludge" phenomena, were also subject to operation.

Dilation of the common bile duct by more than 6 mm was observed in 27% of patients, and signs of stones within the common bile ducts, on average in the population, were found in 16.7%.

Moreover, in patients with asymptomatic cholecystitis, when planning treatment tactics for patients, it is often necessary to consider the condition of the pancreas. The presence of its pathology should alert the surgeon when deciding to perform cholecystectomy, and its consequences need to be considered by the surgeon for the patient, with a confusing clinical picture. According to ultrasound data, the size of the head of the pancreas was, on average, 3.82 ± 1.523 cm, the body – 2.94 ± 0.642 cm, and the tail – 2.97 ± 1.467 cm. These indicators did not go beyond the normal range.

At the same time, in patients with asymptomatic cholecystitis, the pancreas, in many cases, has deviations from the norm. Thus, structural changes indicated unclear and uneven contours of the gland in 64.7% of cases. Smooth contours were visualized in 35.3% of cases, that is, with a frequency of smooth/uneven – 1:3. The density of the pancreas in asymptomatic cholecystitis in 59.9% of observations was hyperechoic.

Isoechoic density was detected in 28.6% of cases of visual control and hypoechoic – in 11.5%. In 4.4% of cases, pseudocysts of the pancreas were diagnosed.

To predict the risk of complications after cholecystectomy in patients, it is important to evaluate the structure of the pancreas. In asymptomatic cholecystitis, pancreatic parenchyma was homogeneous in 35.7% of people and heterogeneous – in 64.3%. In addition, in 18.3% of cases, patients with asymptomatic cholecystitis were found to have calcifications in the parenchyma, and in 7.5%, there were ductal calcifications. Dilation of the Wirsung duct by more than 5 mm was found in 9.5% of patients, while dilation of the lateral ducts by >2 mm was detected in 17.5%.

Thus, the condition of the gallbladder and pancreas in patients with asymptomatic cholecystitis is not normal. Pathological changes in morphology can characterize functional changes in pancreatobiliary interaction. The fragility of the coordinated function of the gallbladder and pancreas can be disrupted by any unjustified cholecystectomy, which is risky for the development of acute and chronic pancreatitis.

In our prospective study to assess the course of asymptomatic cholecystitis in relation to concomitant pathological conditions of the hepatobiliary organs and changes in lipid metabolism, we assigned the leading role to the frequency of detection of postcholecystectomy syndrome. In the studied population of 252 patients, in accordance with the applied management tactics and treatment outcomes, in 103 (40.9%) cases, some patients did not undergo surgical treatment for one reason or another. In 86 (34.1%) patients with asymptomatic cholecystitis, laparoscopic cholecystectomy was performed without complications in the postoperative period. In 63 observations after cholecystectomy for asymptomatic cholecystitis, a clinical picture of the postcholecystectomy syndrome was noted, that is, in 25% of observations. We believe that this is a very high percentage of development of postcholecystectomy syndrome, and we believe a significant change in the tactics of managing patients with asymptomatic cholecystitis in the global sense is necessary. Since our indicators were similar to those of Farthing M. et al. the incidence of post-cholecystectomy clinical complaints was 10-20% of observations [61]. A systematic review by Lamberts M.P. et al. shows that 15-40% of patients experience symptoms after surgery [62]. Studies and clinical guidelines often state that 10-30% of patients experience symptoms after cholecystectomy [63, 64]. Meta-analysis of Latenstein C.S.S et al. confirmed that up to 40% of patients may experience persistent symptoms after surgery [65].

The leading symptoms in 63 patients with postcholecystectomy syndrome were dyspepsia (30.2%), pain (22.2%), and intermittent jaundice (14.3%). The clinically asymptomatic variant, in the absence of complaints against the background of changes in biochemical blood parameters or in the presence of dilatation of the common bile duct of more than 6 mm, was observed in 33.3% of patients. Thus, the variety of clinical manifestations of the postcholecystectomy syndrome in the studied patients actualizes the problem of determining the tactics of treatment of patients with asymptomatic cholecystitis.

Dissatisfaction of patients in the postcholecystectomy period regarding complaints of dyspepsia was associated with nausea (46%), vomiting (3.2%), bitterness in the mouth (30.2%), heartburn (52.4%), belching (44.4%), flatulence (82.5%), constipation (36.5%), loose stools (44.4%). Subsequently, it was revealed that they had a clinical picture of colitis syndrome before the operation, and its correction should be carried out at an early stage, and not after removal of the gallbladder, with pain syndrome.

The presence of signs of postcholecystectomy syndrome of pancreatic or biliary type indicates that the patients were not fully examined. The use of additional criteria for tactics would allow the doctors to postpone cholecystectomy until complete correction of digestive system disorders.

An increase in enzymes in patients with postcholecystectomy syndrome with a clinically asymptomatic variant, in the absence of complaints against the background of changes in biochemical blood parameters, indicates that it continued with the phenomena of hepatosis or hepatodestruction, depending on the degree of liver damage. Thus, cholecystectomy itself not only did not solve the problem of these patients but also, possibly, influenced the aggravation of the parenchyma condition. This is also important to consider when managing such patients since the risk of systemic disorders such as atherosclerosis, hypertension, non-alcoholic fatty liver disease, and renal failure increases. At the same time, cholecystectomy itself did not bring clinical improvement, and anesthesia could cause pathological phenomena in the liver.

We found that indirect signs of the gallbladder condition in asymptomatic cholecystitis depend on the level of lipid metabolism (e.g., **Table 2**). Thus, the lipid accumulation product (LAP, For men: LP = (Waist circumference (cm) – 94) × Triglycerides

Characteristics of the gallbladder	**LAP, cm × mmol/l**	**Atherogenicity coefficient**	**Atherogenic index of plasma (AIP)**	**HOMA-IR index**
Characteristics of the gallbladder				
Volume > avg	16.91 ± 0.269	4.08 ± 1.472	−0.14 ± 0.028	1.84 ± 0.596
Wall thickness > avg	13.67 ± 0.118	3.65 ± 0.748	−0.27 ± 0.013	2.76 ± 0.753
Single polyp	27.68 ± 1.321	2.62 ± 0.521	−0.12 ± 0.084	1.63 ± 0.897
Cholesterosis of gallbladder	24.14 ± 1.789	3.18 ± 1.665	0.56 ± 1.396	2.13 ± 0.529
Low-echo positive suspension (“sludge”)	23.85 ± 1.903	3.09 ± 1.928	0.02 ± 0.015	3.14 ± 0.927
Single stones	21.96 ± 0.872	2.58 ± 0.723	−0.05 ± 0.039	2.84 ± 1.904
Multiple stones	13.83 ± 1.825	3.61 ± 0.281	0.92 ± 0.935	1.97 ± 0.781
Characteristics of the pancreas				
Uneven contours	15.35 ± 0.894	4.12 ± 1.596	0.14 ± 0.024	1.63 ± 0.656
Hyperechoic tissue	14.12 ± 0.286	3.21 ± 0.453	0.17 ± 0.068	2.34 ± 0.653
Heterogeneous structure	25.35 ± 1.993	2.38 ± 0.864	0.12 ± 0.131	1.16 ± 0.687
Parenchyma calcifications	22.16 ± 1.621	3.24 ± 1.017	−0.16 ± 1.346	2.47 ± 0.269
Ductal calcifications	19.74 ± 1.653	3.31 ± 1.642	0.08 ± 0.004	3.04 ± 0.647
Dilation of the lateral ducts>2 мм	17.47 ± 0.849	2.13 ± 0.567	−0.15 ± 0.109	2.16 ± 1.114
Wirsung duct (ductus pancreaticus) >5 мм	14.17 ± 1.647	3.19 ± 0.678	0.11 ± 0.356	1.28 ± 0.029
Pseudocysts of the pancreas	16.49 ± 1.544	4.06 ± 1.323	0.19 ± 0.654	1.13 ± 0.486

Table 2.
The structure of the gallbladder and pancreas depends on the parameters of lipid metabolism with asymptomatic cholecystitis.

(mmol / L); For women: LP = (Waist circumference (cm) – 58) × Triglycerides (mmol / L)), on average in patients with asymptomatic cholecystitis equal to 16.91 ± 0.269 cm × mmol/L, was in correlation with the gallbladder volume, but other indicators were not. The thickness of the gallbladder wall significantly depended on the Atherogenic Index of Plasma (AIP), which was −0.27 ± 0.013 in the study population. Single polyps were most often found with large LAP but low HOMA-IR (Homeostatic Model Assessment of Insulin Resistance) index, on average equal to 1.63 ± 0.897, which is apparently associated with the accumulation and deposition of cholesterol in the body tissues. These patients also had high levels of cholesterol and multiple stones. AIP and Atherogenic Index (AI), equal to 3.61 ± 0.281, on the contrary, were closer to the norm. Thus, it can be said that these indicators are more associated with cholesterol metabolism, rather than with the lithogenicity of bile.

Analyzing the data of patients with asymptomatic cholecystitis, we came to the conclusion that the biochemical composition of bile, as an indicator of the lipid load on the bile ducts, may be a sign of dysfunction of the biliary tract and the deposition of cholesterol in them, causing cholesterosis, dyskinesia, cholestasis, and chronic pancreatitis.

Signs of lipid imbalance in the bile ducts may be secondary changes as a result of pancreatic insufficiency. When assessing pancreatic function, the following dynamics of pancreatic elastase were revealed. The normal ratio was in 6.7% of people, on average equal to 215.62 ± 7.674. Mild exocrine insufficiency was present in 36.5% of cases, with an average level of elastase 162.56 ± 24.678, moderate insufficiency – in 47.6% of observations, and the average level was 124.64 ± 11.754. In 9.1% of cases, severe insufficiency with an average level of pancreatic elastase was detected. 75.71 ± 16.368.

Exocrine insufficiency is indirectly related to gallbladder pathology. It cannot be a clear criterion for the dependence of the development of postcholecystectomy syndrome, which should be taken into account in surgical tactics.

The condition of the pancreas changed in parallel with the lipid spectrum of the blood. When analyzing the lipid metabolism indices, it was revealed that the contours of the pancreas were uneven, with LAP equal to 15.35 ± 0.894. At the same time, the Atherogenic Index did not exceed 4.12 ± 1.596; that is, it was within the normal range. Although AIP was equal to 0.14 ± 0.024, the HOMA-IR index did not exceed 1.63 ± 0.656.

The sign of an uneven contour of the pancreas in ultrasound was not a symptom of lipid metabolism disorder. At the same time, hyperechoic tissue in the pancreas confirms itself as a criterion for lipid metabolism disorder. Moreover, the homogeneous structure of the pancreas was often accompanied by an increase in the LAP level to 25.35 ± 1.993 and a decrease in AI to 2.38 ± 0.864.

In patients with asymptomatic cholecystitis, changes in the pancreas were combined with impaired lipid metabolism. With LAP equal to 15.3 + 0.894 or more ($p = 0.0016$), an uneven contour was more often noted, and there was a combination with calcifications ($p = 0.024$). The heterogeneous structure was often accompanied by an increase in the LAP level to 25.3 + 1.993 ($p = 0.034$) and a decrease in AI to 2.38 + 0.864 ($p = 0.0014$). Dilation of the lateral ducts was accompanied by an increase in LAP to 17.4 + 0.849 ($p = 0.027$), a decrease in AIP -0.15 + 0.109 ($p = 0.017$) and an increase in HOMA-IR index 2.16 + 1.114 ($p = 0.003$).

It is important to note that pseudocysts in patients with asymptomatic cholecystitis were noted to have an increase in the atherogenicity coefficient to 4.06 ± 1.323.

Thus, the ultrasound image of the pancreas, accompanied by heterogeneity of its structure, an increase in the size of the head and body of the pancreas, the presence of calcifications in the parenchyma and ducts, is accompanied by an increase in the frequency and severity of signs of lipid metabolism disorders.

The lipid accumulation index, atherogenic coefficient and atherogenic plasma index may indicate dysfunction of the pancreas, which causes accumulation of low-density lipids. They are released into the bile ducts through impaired bile formation. This is accompanied by accumulation of cholesterol of varying degrees and biliary dyskinesia. That means, a feature of patients with asymptomatic cholecystitis may be pancreatogenic insufficiency, leading to the formation of lipid residues in the bile ducts.

In patients with asymptomatic cholecystitis, visualization of the biliary tract is one of the fundamental criteria for establishing indications for surgical intervention, therefore the clarity and coincidence of the clinical and ultrasound picture will largely determine the likelihood of surgical intervention. However, in patients with asymptomatic cholecystitis, the option with a full normal description of the ultrasound picture occurs only in 38.5% of cases, and visualization difficulties in almost every fifth patient - in 19.8%, which leads to difficulty in establishing indications for surgery or refusal from it. The most reliable signs of the ultrasound picture of biliary tract pathology are “diffuse hyperechogenicity of the liver” and “distal attenuation of the echo signal”.

According to the assessment of biliary tract motility in accordance with the fatty liver disease scales (e.g., **Table 3**), we identified a pattern of hypokinesia with the Non-alcoholic Fatty Liver Disease Liver Fat Score (NLFS) scale indicator – 0.69 ± 0.779, the Fatty Liver Index (FLI) scale – 78.45 ± 1.982, and the Direct

Investigated indicators	**Criteria for liver steatosis, score**		
	NLFS	**DBPTRI**	**FLI**
Liver condition criteria			
Hepatomegaly	0.69 ± 0.375	3.87 ± 1.381	68.3 ± 2.786
Distal echo attenuation	0.79 ± 0.285	4.97 ± 2.046	54.6 ± 1.690
Diffuse hyperechogenicity of the liver (“bright liver”)	0.65 ± 0.385	3.71 ± 1.375	38.5 ± 1.674
Increased echogenicity of the liver compared to the kidneys	0.48 ± 0.286	2.02 ± 1.554	29.4 ± 1.276
Vascular pattern blurring	0.18 ± 0.051	1.89 ± 0.882	41.8 ± 1.965
Criteria for the condition of the biliary tract			
Norm	0.21 ± 0.016	2.23 ± 1.951	25.86 ± 1.583
Dilation of the common bile duct (more 6 мм)	0.66 ± 0.018	2.45 + 1.725	72.43 ± 1.373
Stones within the common bile ducts	0.52 ± 0.194	4.16 ± 1.097	63.25 ± 1.735
Bile duct cysts	0.48 ± 0.236	1.84 ± 0.704	49.71 ± 1.803
The degree of functional state of the biliary tract			
Normokinesis	0.31 ± 0.216	1.64 ± 1.508	18.4 ± 1.598
Hyperkinesis	0.18 ± 0.256	2.97 ± 0.168	24.6 ± 1.642
Hypokinesis of the gallbladder	0.69 ± 0.779	4.28 ± 1.643	78.45 ± 1.982

Table 3.
The state of the bile-producing system in fatty liver with asymptomatic cholecystitis.

Bilirubin to Prothrombin Time Ratio Index (DBPTRI) indicator – 4.28 ± 1.643. At the same time, attention is drawn to the most important laboratory indicators of hepatic steatosis, such as DBPTRI and the FLI scale, accompanied by dilation of the bile ducts and stones in the bile ducts (e.g., **Figure 2**). Thus, the indications for surgery in asymptomatic cholecystitis should be based not only on the ultrasound picture, which is not specific but on a combination of laboratory parameters with ultrasound signs of "distal echo signal attenuation" and "diffuse hyperechogenicity of the liver" (e.g., **Figure 3**).

Based on these indicators, when the patient's clinical picture is unclear, according to ultrasound criteria, it can be assumed that biliary dyskinesia will continue, leading to the phenomena of postcholecystectomy syndrome. In this case, it makes sense to refuse surgical intervention and limit yourself to conservative treatment. It is also possible to conduct corrective therapy after cholecystectomy to restore the normal composition of the lipid spectrum of bile.

Hypokinesia is observed with signs of liver degeneration. Moreover, it is not characteristic of structural changes in the liver itself but is more characteristic of dilation of the bile ducts and stones within the common bile ducts (e.g., **Figure 4**). At the same time, hypokinesia accompanied by an increase in laboratory indicators of liver dystrophy may be the criteria for postponing surgical intervention until the indications for surgical treatment are clear.

In patients with asymptomatic cholecystitis, one of the most common concomitant pathologies is gastrointestinal tract disease. In addition, they often imitate pain syndrome. In some cases, gastrointestinal tract pathology develops after cholecystectomy as a separate nosological picture. We noticed that in patients with asymptomatic cholecystitis, there is a lack of further examination, although there should be a checkup and caution since they are potential patients for the occurrence of postcholecystectomy syndrome.

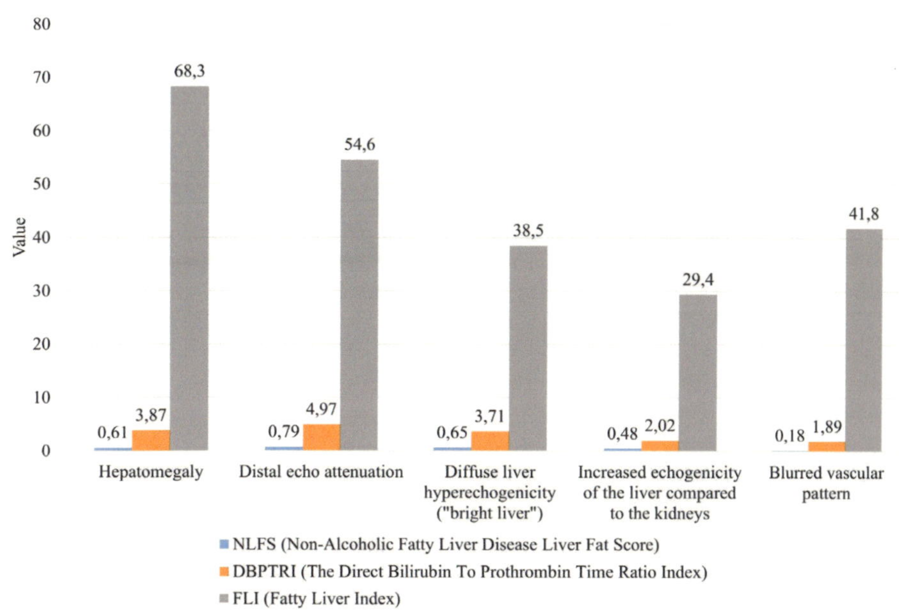

Figure 2.
Ultrasound criteria of the liver for different methods of assessment of steatosis.

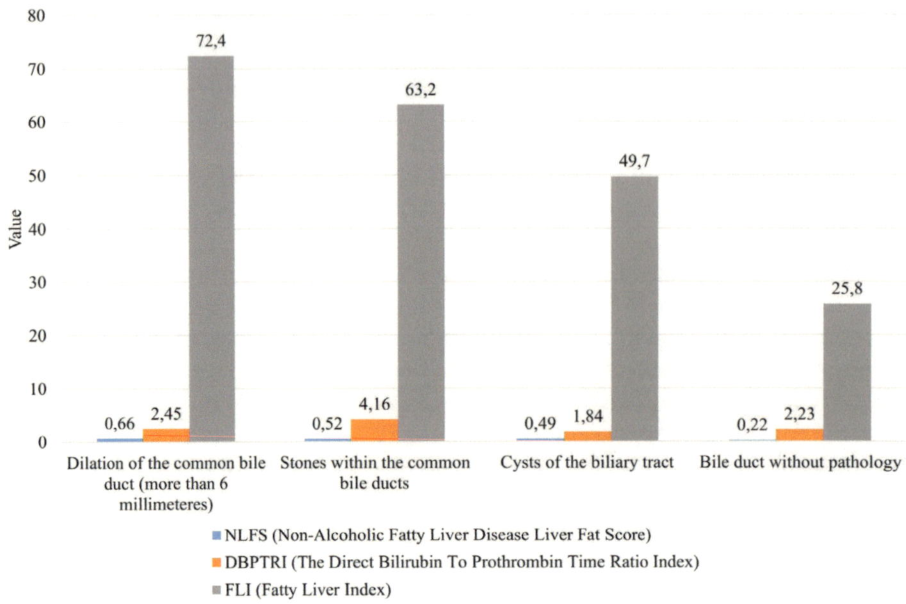

Figure 3.
Ultrasound criteria of the biliary tract with different methods of assessing steatosis.

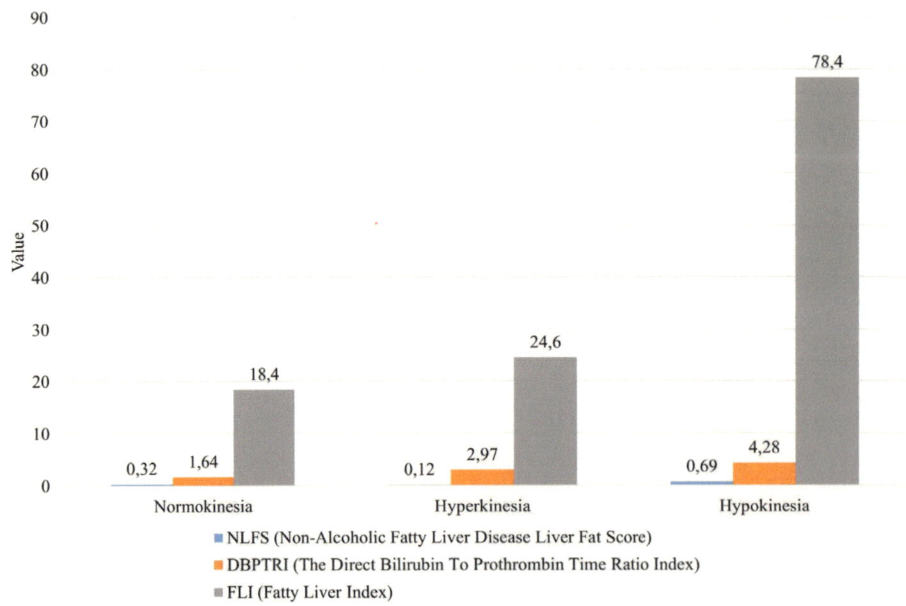

Figure 4.
Functional criteria of the biliary tract for different methods of assessing steatosis.

It is important to note that in patients with asymptomatic cholecystitis, the gallbladder volume above average without gastrointestinal pathology was in 19.4% of patients, with duodenal pathology – in 48.7% of patients, with pathology of the large duodenal papilla – in 47.7% of cases. Thickened gallbladder walls were more often observed in patients with stomach diseases (72.4%) and in patients with pathology of the large duodenal papilla (70.5%). This indicates the presence of signs of not only stagnation but also chronic inflammation in patients with asymptomatic cholecystitis.

Gallbladder cholesterolosis was detected in 41% of patients with duodenal pathology. In patients with stomach and large duodenal papilla diseases, on the contrary, it was the rarest, 14.5% and 9.1% of cases, respectively.

Low-echo positive suspension ("sludge") was more often detected in patients with diseases of the duodenum, in 30.8% of patients, and pathology of the large duodenal papilla – in 29.5%. Single stones were characteristic of patients with diseases of the large duodenal papilla, in 34.1% of cases. Multiple stones, on the contrary, were accompanied by pathology of the stomach, in 61.8% of patients, and the duodenum in 61.5% of people. Thus, preliminary data show that changes in the biliary tract and gallbladder depend not only on the motility of the bile ducts and the composition of bile but also on the morphofunctional state and motility of the upper gastrointestinal tract.

In patients with asymptomatic cholecystitis, it was found that in the entire population, laboratory parameters of lipid metabolism changed taking into account the presence of pathology of the upper gastrointestinal tract. With asymptomatic cholecystitis and without gastrointestinal pathology, the LAP indicator was at the level of 15.76 ± 0.448; this means it exceeded the norm. With gastric pathology, its value was higher and equal to 19.94 ± 0.179, with duodenal diseases, its value was higher and equal to 22.43 ± 0.912, and with biliary-sphincter duodenal (BDS), its value was higher and equal to pathology 24.12 ± 1.789.

The Atherogenic Index was significantly increased in patients with stomach, to an average level of 4.16 ± 1.582, and in patients with BDS – to 3.69 ± 0.141.

In patients with asymptomatic cholecystitis with signs of liver steatosis, the scale level was closer to pathological in case of stomach pathology, as it was equal to 59.65 ± 2.278. At a high level, the FLI scale indicator was 53.79 ± 2.472 for pathology of the large duodenal papilla.

Apparently, in patients with asymptomatic cholecystitis, the lipid profile is not affected by cholecystectomy, but concomitant pathology of the upper gastrointestinal tract contributes to changes in blood composition and dysfunction of the biliary tract of the liver.

An analysis of the frequency of biliary tract motility disorders in patients with asymptomatic cholecystitis showed that in the absence of gastrointestinal pathology, hypokinesia occurs in 70.9%, with gastric pathology – in 63.2%, with duodenal pathology – in 61.6%, in patients with pathology of the large duodenal papilla – in 59.1%.

Thus, the pathology of the upper gastrointestinal tract leads to disorders in the duodenum, especially of inflammatory origin, which is accompanied by duodenostasis and duodenospasm. This increases the risk of postcholecystectomy syndrome in patients with asymptomatic cholecystitis after surgery.

As a result of the above analysis of the influence of upper gastrointestinal pathology on the course of asymptomatic cholecystitis, it can be said that it is the leading link in the development of dyspeptic phenomena based on the dysfunction of the stomach and duodenum by the type of stasis in their lumen, leading to impaired coordination of biliary motility. Against the background of exocrine pancreatic insufficiency, a lithogenic disorder of bile occurs. This is largely due to an increase in intraluminal pressure along the ampulla of the duodenum and an increase in the tone of the sphincter of Oddi. All this, due to intraductal hypertension, inhibits the process of bile secretion, which can be accompanied by a pain syndrome that imitates gallbladder colic in patients with asymptomatic cholecystitis.

This brings the patient to the doctor in order to deal with the symptoms of dyspepsia and pain in the upper abdomen. Against the background of signs of cholestasis, the presence of volumetric formations in the lumen of the gallbladder, and deformation in it, in patients with asymptomatic cholecystitis, erroneous indications for cholecystectomy may be set. Violation of the passage of bile and hepatopancreatoduodenal interaction in patients with asymptomatic cholecystitis is the etiology of dyspepsia, which is important to consider when setting indications for surgical treatment in order to avoid postoperative complications and postcholecystectomy syndrome.

4. Discussion

We consider it important to discuss the existing problems in hepatobiliary surgery on asymptomatic cholecystitis. First of all, we do not claim to have the only correct opinion, and we do not believe that our concept is the truth or dogma. On the contrary, having shared our analysis of literary sources and clinical experience, we believe it is necessary to solve the existing shortcomings in the tactics of managing patients with asymptomatic cholecystitis. This will allow structuring the management of patients, substantiating the indications for cholecystectomy in asymptomatic cholecystitis, reducing the number of unjustified cholecystectomies and financial costs for treatment, and reducing the frequency of complications, primarily postcholecystectomy syndrome.

Thus, on the basis of hepatobiliary surgery, it is necessary to understand the terminology. The concept of "asymptomatic cholecystitis" has the right to exist but requires objective justification and not subjective judgment. Due to the lack of uniformity, the scientific studies that are still carried out on patients with gallbladder stones are fragmented and difficult to compare. Thus, having conducted a literature search in the Pubmed system using several similar definitions that were close in meaning, we identified several directions on this topic. Even more, when discussing the topic being developed among colleagues and editors, we faced the need to clarify mutual understanding for the uniformity of our opinions, and as a result of the discussions, we came to a consensus.

In almost all areas of analysis, the relevance and interest in the topic of asymptomatic cholecystitis has increased in recent years (e.g., **Figure 5**). Thus, in the Pudmed system, when searching for "asymptomatic cholecystitis" we got 500 search results for the criterion "best match". Of course, we understand that different interpretations could

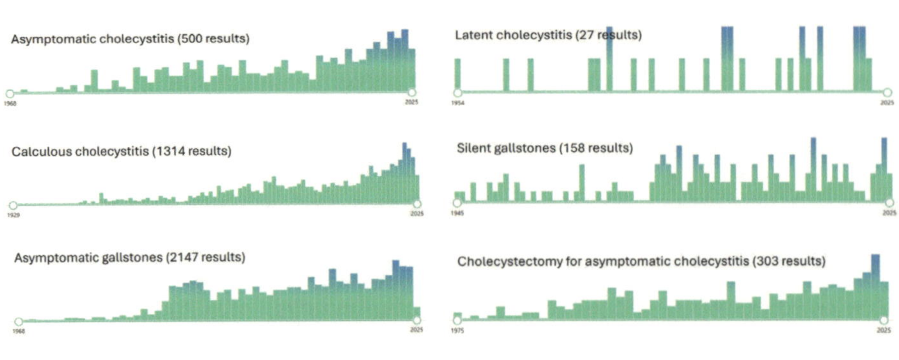

Figure 5.
Frequency of publications about asymptomatic cholecystitis and analogues according to Pubmed search data.

take place, so we also used the term "latent cholecystitis", with which 27 results were found. In 158 papers, the authors indicated "silent gallstones". The most commonly used definitions of gallstones in guidelines and recommendations, and the majority of practicing surgeons are the terms "calculous cholecystitis" – 1314 publications, and "symptomatic gallstones" – 2147 results. As we can see, these two terms define the modern tactics of managing patients with asymptomatic cholecystitis. Our review would be incomplete if we did not take into account the request for "cholecystectomy for asymptomatic cholecystitis", which was found in 303 cases. We also specified the frequency of interest in the terms "asymptomatic chole-lithiasis", "asymptomatic choledocholithiasis", and "cholecystectomy". We did not include them in our analysis because we believe they are of no value to the discussion of the topic of "asymptomatic cholecystitis". However, in the Pudmed system, "asymptomatic choledocholithiasis" was detected 206 times, and "asymptomatic cholelithiasis" was used in 1127 results. For comparison, we would like to mention 45,452 publications for the query "cholecystectomy". This raises many questions and one remarkable conclusion is that most publications on gallstones see the main goal as solving the problem of cholecystectomy as an element of treatment tactics. Shifting the emphasis from the main thing, in our opinion, from the patient to whom indications for surgery are determined.

The problem of disagreement in hepatobiliary surgery is connected precisely with the different goals of consideration in asymptomatic cholecystitis: "cholecystectomy and indications for it" or "the patient and his individual characteristics with the need for surgical treatment".

We would like to repeat that we agree with the clinical recommendations and guidelines of leading societies in Europe and the United States that cholecystectomy is indicated in the presence of gallstones under strict indications. If possible, it should be avoided due to the increased risk due to surgical aggression, even with laparoscopic cholecystectomy, due to anesthesia, due to the high cost of surgical treatment, which is unjustified in asymptomatic cholecystitis. However, we suggest asking the questions differently: "Is gallstone itself a cause of chronic cholecystitis or a consequence of other processes that require correction? Can long-term asymptomatic gallstone itself affect the function of other organs associated with the gallbladder? Can cholecystectomy be one of the stages of complex treatment of patients with abdominal pathology, in whom asymptomatic calculous cholecystitis was the first finding during screening examination?

In the discussion of prophylactic cholecystectomy, we are not its supporters. We believe that preventive removal of the gallbladder is inappropriate for a number of reasons: Firstly, cholecystectomy under the pretext of "risk of complications" preserves the possibility of intra- and postoperative complications, so it is illogical to do so. Secondly, removing an organ with potentially dangerous complications is unethical. Thirdly, performing a surgical operation to resect a "sick organ" without attempting conservative treatment is inhumane.

Based on our above clinical analysis of patients with asymptomatic cholecystitis, we would like to propose a surgical tactic that will take into account most interests and solve a range of problems in treatment.

Basically, we consider a patient with asymptomatic cholecystitis who learned about the gallbladder during an ultrasound or other examination, but before that, he had no complaints and symptoms from the abdominal organs, or he was bothered by a number of vague manifestations similar to the signs of gallstone disease. Of course, a dilemma arises – surgery or not? A solution can be seen with the use of preventive planning tactics for asymptomatic cholecystitis or PPTACh, presented in **Figure 6**.

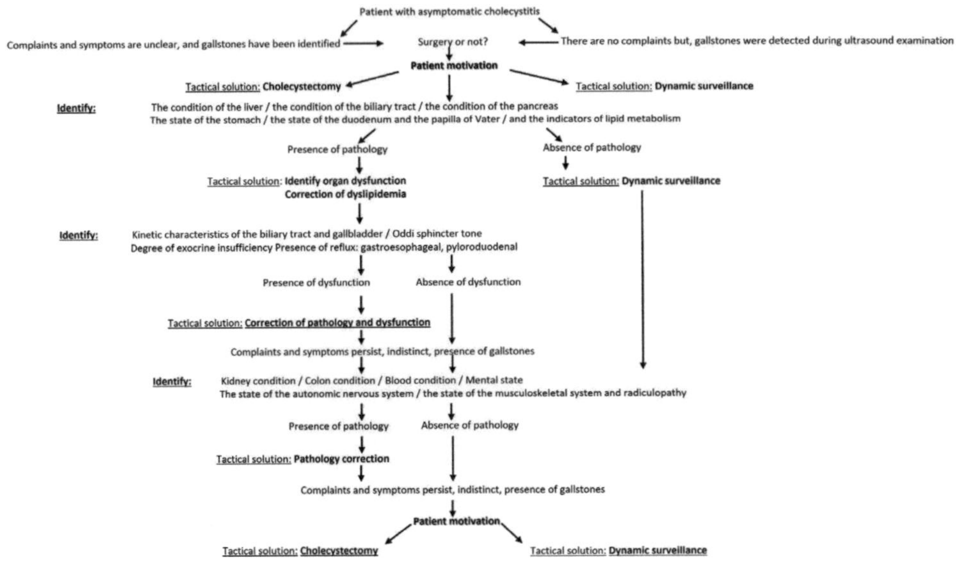

Figure 6.
Preventive planning tactics in the management of patients with asymptomatic cholecystitis.

The priority is to find out the patient's opinion on this matter, his quality of life, and his needs that we could allow him to realize with our recommendations. Naturally, this problem has three solutions: at first glance, it seems that cholecystectomy or dynamic observation are the most acceptable options. They are currently the most popular and accepted as the main option in the treatment of patients with asymptomatic cholecystitis. But as practice shows, the frequency of postcholecystectomy syndrome in this case is 1:4, or 25% of the population. At the same time, it is important to note that in hepatobiliary surgery, we still do not consider several more factors: the frequency of simultaneous operations with cholecystectomy for stone disease, as well as how many patients are treated by gastroenterologists and therapists for other diagnoses, but have asymptomatic cholecystitis, and what are the results of this treatment. Therefore, we see the third direction of development and option as the leading one: justification of the involvement of asymptomatic cholecystitis in other organs, as well as a departure from the subjective judgment of the surgeon and the opinion of the patient with the objectification of indications for cholecystectomy.

On the way to solving the dilemma of "surgery or not?" we propose an algorithm for preventive planning tactics for asymptomatic cholecystitis and we call it PPTACh. PPTACh includes an examination to clarify the involvement of adjacent organs of the hepatobiliarypancreatoduodenal zone in the pathological process called "asymptomatic cholecystitis". The conditions of the liver, bile ducts, pancreas, stomach, and duodenum with the Vater's papilla revealed. Also, for cholelithiasis, it is pathogenetically necessary to evaluate the lipid spectrum and fat metabolism in the body. In the absence of pathology in these organs with asymptomatic cholecystitis, it is necessary to continue the examination to determine the condition of the kidneys, colon, blood, and hematopoiesis, the state of the nervous system, especially the autonomic (sympathetic and parasympathetic), the state of the musculoskeletal system, especially the spine and the presence of radiculopathy, as well as the mental status of the patient, which can determine his lifestyle and habits.

Detection of the pathology of the organs of the hepatobiliarypancreatoduodenal zone requires an assessment of their function since the treatment of this pathology is not only surgical but mostly pathogenetic conservative. The scope of the examination is determined individually for each patient but may include the kinetic characteristics of the biliary tract and the tone of the sphincter of Oddi, the degree of exocrine pancreatic insufficiency, and the severity of gastroesophageal or pyloroduodenal reflux. In the presence of pathology and dysfunction of any organ in a patient with asymptomatic cholecystitis, it is necessary to treat such patients with correction of internal systems.

At the same time, regardless of the presence of pathology of the organs of the hepatobiliarypancreatoduodenal zone, all patients with asymptomatic cholecystitis, as well as without disorders, need to analyze the condition of the kidneys, colon, blood, and hematopoiesis, assess sympathetic and parasympathetic nervous systems, the state of the musculoskeletal system, as well as the mental status of the patient. This will exclude their omission in preoperative planning or when choosing therapeutic tactics.

Patients with asymptomatic cholecystitis who have undergone a course of complex treatment for the identified pathology or after justifying its exclusion can re-evaluate their motivation for a particular treatment choice. In this case, the doctor will have answers to the following questions: "Is gallstone itself a cause of chronic cholecystitis or a consequence of other processes that require correction? Can long-term asymptomatic gallstone itself affect the function of other organs associated with the gallbladder? Can cholecystectomy be one of the stages of complex treatment of patients with abdominal pathology, in whom asymptomatic calculous cholecystitis was the first finding during a screening examination? Thus, arguments based on facts appear when choosing surgical tactics with decisions: performing cholecystectomy or dynamic observation.

On the one hand, the proposed tactics look routine, labor-intensive, and costly, but it is pathogenetically justified in asymptomatic cholecystitis. This does not greatly exceed the financial costs compared to modern surgical treatment. The advantage of the proposed tactics is patient routing and targeted combined treatment, where each stage is reasoned, and cholecystectomy is an element in an integrated approach and has its own surgical value and role in preventing complications.

5. Conclusions

As a result of the above, the following conclusion can be made: the frequency and severity of gallbladder pathology in patients with asymptomatic cholecystitis are due to the disturbance of cholesterol metabolism and the lipid spectrum of bile. This is largely due not to exocrine pancreatic insufficiency, the signs of which in patients with asymptomatic cholecystitis are found chaotically.

But to a greater extent, it is associated with the peculiarities of the anatomical structure of the gallbladder, which in a quarter of cases is characterized by small size, bending, dysfunction, and biliary dyskinesia against the background of thickening of bile. The development of exocrine insufficiency and impaired passage of bile directly in the biliary tract can be conditions for the deposition of fat droplets in the mucous membrane, thereby maintaining dyskinesia and cholestasis. This increases the risk of the formation not of cholesterol stones or polyps in the gallbladder but of the lithogenic properties of bile, which can subsequently form bilirubin or calcified stones. One of the criteria for confirming a violation of the excretory function of bile is pancreatic dysfunction, which is, among other things, secondary. At the same time, it maintains calcification and pseudocysts in the parenchyma of the pancreas, accompanied by an increase in the head of the pancreas and body size. This is all against the background of asymptomatic cholecystitis in the absence of an obvious clinical picture of chronic pancreatitis, which is a latent form of organ dysfunction in the hepatoduodenal zone.

These changes, of course, can be considered criteria as indications and contraindications for surgical treatment in patients with asymptomatic cholecystitis. But gallbladder dysfunction in this situation can be aggravated by exocrine pancreatic insufficiency, therefore, its assessment is important in treatment tactics. Apparently, with a mild form of exocrine insufficiency, it most likely makes sense to perform surgical intervention, since it allows for the preservation of pancreatic function, which has a beneficial effect on the composition of bile.

As a result, in this chapter devoted to the situation around "asymptomatic cholecystitis" and strategies for managing such patients, we would like to note that although this disease exists, approaches to its study vary, and attempts are rare and multidirectional. As a result, today's practice in hepatobiliary surgery limits preoperative diagnostics, ignoring the secondary nature (i.e., the result of another pathological process in the body) of stone formation in a patient with asymptomatic cholecystitis. Cholecystectomy performed in this way for asymptomatic cholecystitis often does not solve the treatment issues but obscures the true cause of the complaints. A number of tactical errors lead to the continued risk of developing postcholecystectomy syndrome and blurring useful recommendations for managing such patients. A detailed analysis of each stage of the tactical search in patients with asymptomatic cholecystitis will provide a new approach to biliary tract surgery and solve this problem.

6. Key messages

- Asymptomatic cholecystitis is a pathological process in the gallbladder, accompanied by the formation of stones, polyps, and cholesterosis, which is a reflection of the pathology and dysfunction of many organs and systems.

- Asymptomatic cholecystitis has a clinical course, but the complaints and symptoms are unclear because they are not similar to cystic colic; they can be disguised as a clinical picture of diseases of other organs or be hidden due to a more pronounced manifestation of related pathology, therefore, a careful chronological analysis of the medical history is required.

- A comprehensive step-by-step sequential examination of a patient with asymptomatic cholecystitis should become a key link in surgical tactics for choosing treatment.

- Most importantly, in patients with asymptomatic cholecystitis, preventive planning tactics (PPTACh) in diagnostics and treatment are a necessity to identify indications for surgery, reduce surgical risks, avoid postoperative complications, and prevent the development of postcholecystectomy syndrome. It must be noted that prophylactic cholecystitisectomy is not recommended at all.

- Cholecystitisectomy is a pathogenetically justified operation for asymptomatic cholecystitis only if its effect on other organs and the body as a whole is proven.
- Cholecystitisectomy for asymptomatic cholecystitis should be considered as an additional or simultaneous stage in the complex treatment of the patient.
- Dynamic observation, including postoperative, for asymptomatic cholecystitis should be carried out under the supervision of a gastroenterologist and therapist, who will need to involve a surgeon at any time to adjust the treatment.

Acknowledgements

The authors express their gratitude to the leadership of Sechenov University for the opportunity to conduct clinical research and engage in scientific research.

Conflict of interest

The authors do not have any financial or legal conflicts of interest. The manuscript was compiled taking into account one's own opinion on the problems without claiming someone else's intellectual property. The work was carried out on the basis of Sechenov University without financial costs and investments.

Author details

Sergey Yurievich Muraviev* and Mehrshad Ebrahimnezhad
Federal State Autonomous Educational Institution of Higher Education "I.M. Sechenov First Moscow State Medical University" of the Ministry of Health of the Russian Federation (Sechenov University), Moscow, Russia

*Address all correspondence to: sechhospitalsurgery@gmail.com

References

[1] Virk S, Arora H, Patil P, Sarang B, Khajanchi M, Bains L, et al. An Indian surgeon's perspective on management of asymptomatic gallstones. Asian Journal of Endoscopic Surgery. 2024;**17**(2):e13297. DOI: 10.1111/ases.13297

[2] Abraham S, Rivero HG, Erlikh IV, Griffith LF, Kondamudi VK. Surgical and nonsurgical management of gallstones. American Family Physician. 2014;**89**(10):795-802

[3] Schirmer BD, Winters KL, Edlich RF. Cholelithiasis and cholecystitis. Journal of Long-Term Effects of Medical Implants. 2005;**15**(3):329-338. DOI: 10.1615/jlongtermeffmedimplants.v15.i3.90

[4] Patel N, Jensen KK, Shaaban AM, Korngold E, Foster BR. Multimodality imaging of cholecystectomy complications. Radiographics. 2022;**42**(5):1303-1319. DOI: 10.1148/rg.210106

[5] National Institute for Health and Care Excellence (NICE). National Institute for Health and Care Excellence: Guidelines [Internet]. London: National Institute for Health and Care Excellence (NICE); 2003. Available from: https://www.ncbi.nlm.nih.gov/books/NBK11822/ [Accessed: October 7, 2024]

[6] Manes G, Paspatis G, Aabakken L, Anderloni A, Arvanitakis M, Ah-Soune P, et al. Endoscopic management of common bile duct stones: European Society of Gastrointestinal Endoscopy (ESGE) guideline. Endoscopy. 2019;**51**(5):472-491. DOI: 10.1055/a-0862-0346

[7] Chapman MH, Thorburn D, Hirschfield GM, Webster GGJ, Rushbrook SM, Alexander G, et al. British Society of Gastroenterology and UK-PSC guidelines for the diagnosis and management of primary sclerosing cholangitis. Gut. 2019;**68**(8):1356-1378. DOI: 10.1136/gutjnl-2018-317993

[8] European Association for the Study of the Liver (EASL). EASL clinical practice guidelines on the prevention, diagnosis and treatment of gallstones. Journal of Hepatology. 2016;**65**(1):146e181. DOI: 10.1016/j.jhep.2016.03.005

[9] Kiriyama S, Kozaka K, Takada T, Strasberg SM, Pitt HA, Gabata T, et al. Tokyo guidelines 2018: Diagnostic criteria and severity grading of acute cholangitis (with videos). Journal of Hepato-Biliary-Pancreatic Sciences. 2018;**25**(1):17-30. DOI: 10.1002/jhbp.512

[10] European Society of Gastrointestinal Endoscopy (ESGE), European Association for the Study of the Liver (EASL). ESGE and EASL Clinical Guideline [Internet]. European Society of Gastrointestinal Endoscopy (ESGE), European Association for the Study of the Liver (EASL). 2025;**57**:166-185. DOI: 10.1055/a-2481-7048. Available from: https://www.easl.eu/ [Accessed: May 12, 2024]

[11] American College of Gastroenterology (ACG). ACG Guideline on Gallstone Disease [Internet]. American College of Gastroenterology (ACG). Columbus, OH: Royce Groce, MD, Ohio State University; 2021. Available from: https://gi.org/topics/gallstones-in-women/ [Accessed: November 17, 2024]

[12] UpToDate. Approach to the Patient With Incidental Gallstones [Internet]. 2023. Available from: https://www.uptodate.com/ [Accessed: October 7, 2024]

[13] Kusano T, Isa T, Ohtsubo M, Yasaka T, Furukawa M. Natural progression of untreated hepatolithiasis that shows no clinical signs at its initial presentation. Journal of Clinical Gastroenterology. 2001;**33**(2):114-117. DOI: 10.1097/00004836-200108000-00004

[14] Chen JW, Thomas A, Woods CM, Schloithe AC, Toouli J, Saccone GT. Sphincter of Oddi dysfunction produces acute pancreatitis in the possum. Gut. 2000;**47**(4):539-545. DOI: 10.1136/gut.47.4.539

[15] Xu XD, Qian JQ, Dai JJ, Sun ZX. Endoscopic treatment for choledocholithiasis in asymptomatic patients. Journal of Gastroenterology and Hepatology. 2020;**35**(1):165-169. DOI: 10.1111/jgh.14790

[16] Lee BJH, Yap QV, Low JK, Chan YH, Shelat VG. Cholecystectomy for asymptomatic gallstones: Markov decision tree analysis. World Journal of Clinical Cases. 2022;**10**(29):10399-10412. DOI: 10.12998/wjcc.v10.i29.10399

[17] Alves JR, Klock DM, Ronzani FG, Santos SLD, Amico EC. Asymptomatic cholelithiasis: Expectant or cholecystectomy. A systematic review. Arquivos Brasileiros de Cirurgia Digestiva. 2023;**36**:e1747. DOI: 10.1590/0102-672020230029e1747

[18] Sebghatollahi V, Parsa M, Minakari M, Azadbakht S. A clinician's guide to gallstones and common bile duct (CBD): A study protocol for a systematic review and evidence-based recommendations. Health Science Reports. 2023;**6**(9):e1555. DOI: 10.1002/hsr2.1555

[19] Fujita N, Yasuda I, Endo I, Isayama H, Iwashita T, Ueki T, et al. Evidence-based clinical practice guidelines for cholelithiasis 2021. Journal of Gastroenterology. 2023;**58**(9):801-833. DOI: 10.1007/s00535-023-02014-6

[20] Hakuta R, Hamada T, Nakai Y, Oyama H, Kanai S, Suzuki T, et al. Natural history of asymptomatic bile duct stones and association of endoscopic treatment with clinical outcomes. Journal of Gastroenterology. 2020;**55**(1):78-85. DOI: 10.1007/s00535-019-01612-7

[21] Kamaya A, Fung C, Szpakowski JL, Fetzer DT, Walsh AJ, Alimi Y, et al. Management of incidentally detected gallbladder polyps: Society of radiologists in ultrasound consensus conference recommendations. Radiology. 2022;**305**(2):277-289. DOI: 10.1148/radiol.213079

[22] Kumar S, Kurian N, Singh RK, Chidipotu VR, Kumar S, Raj AK, et al. Surgical management of cystic duct stump calculi causing post-cholecystectomy syndrome: A prospective study. Journal of Minimal Access Surgery. 2023;**19**(2):257-262. DOI: 10.4103/jmas.jmas_75_22

[23] Chandra R, Liddle RA. Recent advances in the regulation of pancreatic secretion. Current Opinion in Gastroenterology. 2014;**30**(5):490-494. DOI: 10.1097/MOG.0000000000000099

[24] Rehfeld JF. Cholecystokinin and the hormone concept. Endocrine Connections. 2021;**10**(3):R139-R150. DOI: 10.1530/EC-21-0025

[25] Sayin SI, Wahlström A, Felin J, Jäntti S, Marschall H, Bamberg K, et al. Gut microbiota regulates bile acid metabolism by reducing the levels of tauro-beta-muricholic acid, a naturally occurring FXR antagonist. Cell Metabolism. 2013;**17**(2):225-235. DOI: 10.1016/j.cmet.2013.01.003

[26] Ridlon JM, Kang DJ, Hylemon PB, Bajaj JS. Bile acids and the gut microbiome. Current Opinion in Gastroenterology. 2014;**30**(3):332-338. DOI: 10.1097/MOG.0000000000000057

[27] Lee H, Askar A, Makanji D, Ranjha K, Karki BB, Courcol J, et al. The incidence of post cholecystectomy pain (PCP) syndrome at 12 months following laparoscopic cholecystectomy: A prospective evaluation in 200 patients. Scandinavian Journal of Pain. 2024;**24**(1):20230067. DOI: 10.1515/sjpain-2023-0067

[28] Hall L, Halle-Smith J, Evans R, Toogood G, Wiggins T, Markar SR, et al. Ursodeoxycholic acid in the management of symptomatic gallstone disease: Systematic review and clinician survey. BJS Open. 2023;7(2):zrac152. DOI: 10.1093/bjsopen/zrac152

[29] Agarwal DK, Choudhuri G, Saraswat VA, Negi TS, Kapoor VK, Saxena R. Duodenal bile examination in identifying potential non-responders to bile salt treatment and its comparison with gall bladder bile examination. Gut. 1994;**35**(1):112-116. DOI: 10.1136/gut.35.1.112

[30] Jones MW, Weir CB, Ghassemzadeh S. Gallstones (Cholelithiasis). Treasure Island (FL): StatPearls Publishing; 2025. Available from: https://www.ncbi.nlm.nih.gov/books/NBK459370/ [Accessed: January 16, 2025]

[31] Cotton PB, Elta GH, Carter CR, Pasricha PJ, Corazziari ES. Rome IV. Gallbladder and sphincter of Oddi disorders. Gastroenterology. 2016;**150**:1420-1429. DOI: 10.1053/j.gastro.2016.02.033

[32] Luu MB, Deziel DJ. Unusual complications of gallstones. The Surgical Clinics of North America. 2014;**94**(2):377-394. DOI: 10.1016/j.suc.2014.01.002

[33] Corazziari E, Attili AF, Angeletti C, De Santis A. Gallstones, cholecystectomy and irritable bowel syndrome (IBS) MICOL population-based study. Digestive and Liver Disease. 2008;**40**(12):944-950. DOI: 10.1016/j.dld.2008.02.013

[34] Murshid KR. Asymptomatic gallstones: Should we operate? Saudi Journal of Gastroenterology. 2007;**13**(2):57-69. DOI: 10.4103/1319-3767.32179

[35] Larabi AB, Masson HLP, Bäumler AJ. Bile acids as modulators of gut microbiota composition and function. Gut Microbes. 2023;**15**(1):2172671. DOI: 10.1080/19490976.2023.2172671

[36] Liwinski T, Heinemann M, Schramm C. The intestinal and biliary microbiome in autoimmune liver disease-current evidence and concepts. Seminars in Immunopathology. 2022;**44**(4):485-507. DOI: 10.1007/s00281-022-00936-6

[37] Song ST, Cai LY, Zeng X, Xie WF. Gut microbial profile in asymptomatic gallstones. Frontiers in Microbiology. 2022;**13**:882265. DOI: 10.3389/fmicb.2022.882265

[38] Wu T, Zhang Z, Liu B, Hou D, Liang Y, Zhang J, et al. Gut microbiota dysbiosis and bacterial community assembly associated with cholesterol gallstones in large-scale study. BMC Genomics. 2013;**14**:669. DOI: 10.1186/1471-2164-14-669

[39] Frost F, Kacprowski T, Rühlemann M, Weiss S, Bang C, Franke A, et al. Carrying asymptomatic gallstones is not associated with changes in intestinal microbiota composition and diversity but cholecystectomy with significant dysbiosis. Scientific Reports.

2021;**11**(1):6677. DOI: 10.1038/s41598-021-86247-6

[40] Ahmed MH, Barakat S, Almobarak AO. The association between renal stone disease and cholesterol gallstones: The easy to believe and not hard to retrieve theory of the metabolic syndrome. Renal Failure. 2014;**36**(6):957-962. DOI: 10.3109/0886022X.2014.900424

[41] Taylor EN, Chan AT, Giovannucci EL, Curhan GC. Cholelithiasis and the risk of nephrolithiasis. The Journal of Urology. 2011;**186**(5):1882-1887. DOI: 10.1016/j.juro.2011.06.067

[42] Kulaçoğlu H, Dener C, Kama NA. Urinary retention after elective cholecystectomy. American Journal of Surgery. 2001;**182**(3):226-229. DOI: 10.1016/s0002-9610(01)00703-6

[43] Nagorni EA, Kouklakis G, Tsaroucha A, Foutzitzi S, Courcoutsakis N, Romanidis K, et al. Post-laparoscopic cholecystectomy Mirizzi syndrome induced by polymeric surgical clips: A case report and review of the literature. Journal of Medical Case Reports. 2016;**10**:135. DOI: 10.1186/s13256-016-0932-5

[44] Chae MS, Kravchuk OA. Point of care ultrasound in rapid diagnosis of acute cholangitis and emphysematous cholecystitis: A case report. International Journal of Emergency Medicine. 2025;**18**(1):29. DOI: 10.1186/s12245-025-00823-5

[45] Portincasa P, Di Ciaula A, Bonfrate L, Stella A, Garruti G, Lamont JT. Metabolic dysfunction-associated gallstone disease: Expecting more from critical care manifestations. Internal and Emergency Medicine. 2023;**18**(7):1897-1918. DOI: 10.1007/s11739-023-03355-z

[46] Behari A, Kapoor VK. Asymptomatic gallstones (AsGS) - to treat or not to? The Indian Journal of Surgery. 2012;**74**(1):4-12. DOI: 10.1007/s12262-011-0376-5

[47] Morimoto M, Matsuo T, Mori N. Management of porcelain gallbladder, its risk factors, and complications: A review. Diagnostics (Basel). 2021;**11**(6):1073. DOI: 10.3390/diagnostics11061073

[48] Goel A, Agarwal A, Gupta S, Bhagat TS, Kumar G, Gupta AK. Porcelain gallbladder. Euroasian Journal of Hepatogastroenterology. 2017;**7**(2):181-182. DOI: 10.5005/jp-journals-10018-1244

[49] Geller SA, Campos FPF. Porcelain gallbladder. Autopsy and Case Reports [Internet]. 2015;**5**(4):5-7. DOI: 10.4322/acr.2015.024

[50] Kwon AH, Inui H, Matsui Y, Uchida Y, Hukui J, Kamiyama Y. Laparoscopic cholecystectomy in patients with porcelain gallbladder based on the preoperative ultrasound findings. Hepato-Gastroenterology. 2004;**51**(58):950-953

[51] DesJardins H, Duy L, Scheirey C, Schnelldorfer T. Porcelain gallbladder: Is observation a safe option in select populations? Journal of the American College of Surgeons. 2018;**226**(6):1064-1069. DOI: 10.1016/j.jamcollsurg.2017.11.026

[52] Gutt C, Schläfer S, Lammert F. The treatment of gallstone disease. Deutsches Ärzteblatt International. 2020;**117**(9):148-158. DOI: 10.3238/arztebl.2020.0148

[53] Mc Geehan G, Melly C, O'Connor N, Bass G, Mohseni S, Bucholc M, et al. Prophylactic cholecystectomy offers best outcomes following ERCP clearance of common bile duct stones: A meta-analysis.

European Journal of Trauma and Emergency Surgery. 2023;**49**(5):2257-2267. DOI: 10.1007/s00068-022-02070-2

[54] Bekkali NL, Oppong KW. How to manage postcholecystectomy abdominal pain. Frontline Gastroenterology. 2019;**12**(2):145-150. DOI: 10.1136/flgastro-2019-101190

[55] Duncan CB, Riall TS. Evidence-based current surgical practice: Calculous gallbladder disease. Journal of Gastrointestinal Surgery. 2012;**16**(11):2011-2025. DOI: 10.1007/s11605-012-2024-1

[56] Russian Society of Surgeons (or relevant association). Russian Clinical Guidelines for Cholecystitis [Internet]. Russia: Russian Society of Surgeons (or relevant association); 2024. Available from: https://endoexpert.ru/dokumenty-i-prikazy/krkholetsistit/ [Accessed: April 15, 2025]

[57] Wysocki AP, Allen J, Rey-Conde T, North JB. Analysis of deficiencies in care following cholecystectomy. Journal of Visceral Surgery. 2015;**152**(4):217-222. DOI: 10.1016/j.jviscsurg.2015.06.008

[58] Ahmed I, Hudson J, Innes K, Hernández R, Gillies K, Bruce R, et al. Effectiveness of conservative management versus laparoscopic cholecystectomy in the prevention of recurrent symptoms and complications in adults with uncomplicated symptomatic gallstone disease (C-GALL trial): Pragmatic, multicentre randomised controlled trial. BMJ. 2023;**383**:e075383. DOI: 10.1136/bmj-2023-075383

[59] Park S, Jeong S, Park SJ, Song J, Kim SM, Chang J, et al. Associations of cholecystectomy with metabolic health changes and incident cardiovascular disease: A retrospective cohort study. Scientific Reports. 2024;**14**(1):3195. DOI: 10.1038/s41598-024-53161-6

[60] Tint GS, Salen G, Colalillo A, Graber D, Verga D, Speck J, et al. Ursodeoxycholic acid: A safe and effective agent for dissolving cholesterol gallstones. Annals of Internal Medicine. 1982;**97**(3):351-356. DOI: 10.7326/0003-4819-97-3-351

[61] Farthing M, Roberts SE, Samuel DG, Williams JG, Thorne K, Morrison-Rees S, et al. Survey of digestive health across Europe: Final report. Part 1: The burden of gastro-intestinal diseases and the organisation and delivery of gastroenterology services across Europe. United European. Gastroenterologisches Journal. 2014;**2**(6):539-543. DOI: 10.1177/2050640614554154

[62] Lamberts MP, Lugtenberg M, Rovers MM, Roukema AJ, Drenth JP, Westert GP, et al. Persistent and de novo symptoms after cholecystectomy: A systematic review of cholecystectomy effectiveness. Surgical Endoscopy. 2013;**27**(3):709-718. DOI: 10.1007/s00464-012-2516-9

[63] Lundgren L, Muszynska C, Ros A, Persson G, Gimm O, Valter L, et al. Are incidental gallbladder cancers missed with a selective approach of gallbladder histology at cholecystectomy? World Journal of Surgery. 2018;**42**(4):1092-1099. DOI: 10.1007/s00268-017-4215-0

[64] Bisgaard T, Klarskov B, Rosenberg J, Kehlet H. Characteristics and prediction of early pain after laparoscopic cholecystectomy. Pain. 2001;**90**(3):261-269. DOI: 10.1016/S0304-3959(00)00406-1

[65] Latenstein CSS, Wennmacker SZ, de Jong JJ, van Laarhoven CJHM, Drenth JPH, de Reuver PR. Etiologies of long-term postcholecystectomy symptoms: A systematic review. Gastroenterology Research and Practice. 2019;**2019**:4278373. DOI: 10.1155/2019/4278373

Chapter 3

Imaging of Biliary Tree

Tsvetelina Teneva and Aleksandar Zlatarov

Abstract

Biliary imaging includes different techniques, starting with ultrasound as the first-line imaging modality of choice, then the cross-sectional or tomography imaging—computed tomography and magnetic resonance imaging, ending with invasive procedures as endoscopic retrograde cholangiography and percutaneous transhepatic cholangiography. Positron-emission tomography scan and endosonography are additional imaging studies to be mentioned. In this chapter, the imaging approach is discussed according to different clinical scenarios. Jaundice is the most common biliary/liver disease, and the most important question imaging has to answer is whether the icterus is obstructive or non-obstructive. Which imaging methods would define the biliary tree pathology as indicated for surgical treatment is another important question. Diagnostic pathways in biliary colic and acute cholecystitis are discussed. Sonographic Murphy's sign, gallstones, and pericholecystic fluid are important imaging findings. Choledocholithiasis and cholangitis are key findings on ultrasound, computed tomography, and magnetic resonance cholangiopancreatography. Cholangiocarcinoma is the cancer deriving from the biliary structures. It has different types, and in many cases, it is radiographically indistinguishable from hepatocellular carcinoma and even from benign tumors of liver and biliary tree. Imaging hallmarks on computed tomography and magnetic resonance imaging, especially on contrast-enhanced techniques, should be taken into consideration. Lastly are included post-surgical and iatrogenic biliary injuries such as bile leak and bilomas. Not on focus in this chapter are some special considerations—pediatric and congenital biliary disorders, biliary atresia, choledochal cysts, liver transplantation, and biliary imaging, pre- and post-transplant complications. Emerging technologies and future directions, especially artificial intelligence in biliary imaging, are also excluded.

Keywords: biliary tree, imaging, ultrasound, CT, MRCP, ERCP, PTC, jaundice, biloma, bile leak, cholecystectomy

1. Introduction

The biliary tree and gallbladder play crucial roles in the digestion and absorption of lipids, as well as in the excretion of waste products from the liver. The biliary tree consists of a network of ducts that transport bile, including the intrahepatic hepatic ducts and the extrahepatic ducts—the anterior duct (ductus anterior), posterior duct (ductus posterior), medial duct (ductus medialis), and lateral duct (ductus lateralis)—the right and left hepatic ducts (ductus hepaticus dexter, ductus hepaticus sinister), common hepatic duct (ductus hepaticus communis), cystic duct (ductus cysticus), and common bile duct (ductus choledochus), which excretes the bile into duodenum trough the ampulla of Vater.

Disorders of the biliary tree and gallbladder can lead to significant morbidity. Common conditions such as gallstones, cholecystitis, and cholangitis can disrupt the flow of bile, causing pain, infection, and potential complications such as pancreatitis or biliary obstruction. This chapter aims to review the imaging modalities for the biliary tree and gallbladder, highlighting common diseases and their management.

2. Clinical presentation and imaging approach in different clinical scenarios

2.1 Jaundice

Obstructive jaundice results from a blockage in the bile ducts, preventing bile from flowing from the liver to the intestines. It is characterized by direct hyperbilirubinemia and elevated cholestasis enzymes. Common causes include bile duct stones, tumors, and strictures [1].

Non-obstructive jaundice is often due to liver diseases such as hepatitis or metabolic disorders, and it is characterized by indirect hyperbilirubinemia.

To differentiate obstructive jaundice from non-obstructive jaundice, several clinical, biochemical, and imaging criteria are used, as described in **Table 1**.

Imaging techniques for biliary tree in the setting of obstructive icterus aim at detecting the obstruction, the level of dilation of biliary tree- intra- and/or extrahepatic and respectively the diameter of dilated ducts.

Ultrasonography (USG) is often the first imaging modality; it can detect bile duct dilation and stones with high sensitivity and specificity [2]. However, it may not always identify the exact cause or extent of obstruction.

Magnetic resonance cholangiopancreatography (MRCP), as a non-invasive imaging technique, provides detailed images of the biliary and pancreatic ducts and is superior to USG in identifying the cause and extent of obstruction [2].

Endoscopic retrograde cholangiopancreatography (ERCP): This invasive procedure is used both diagnostically and therapeutically to visualize and treat obstructions in the bile ducts.

Criteria	Obstructive jaundice	Non-obstructive jaundice
Bilirubin type	Direct hyperbilirubinemia	Indirect hyperbilirubinemia
Common causes	Bile duct stones, tumors, and strictures	Hepatitis, metabolic disorders
Imaging	Primary biliary tree-focused imaging: US, MRCP, ERCP	Primary liver-focused imaging: CT, MRI,
Contrast-enhanced techniques	+/−	+++
Treatment	Surgical/endoscopic relief of obstruction	Treat the underlying liver disease

Table 1.
Laboratory, imaging, and clinical criteria for obstructive and non-obstructive jaundice.

2.1.1 Management and treatment

Treatment in obstructive jaundice often involves relieving the obstruction through surgical or endoscopic procedures. For benign causes like stones, endoscopic removal or laparoscopic surgery is common. Malignant causes may require major surgical resections or palliative stenting [3].

Management in non-obstructive jaundice focuses on treating the underlying liver disease, such as antiviral therapy for hepatitis or supportive care for metabolic disorders.

2.2 Benign biliary obstruction

The choice of imaging method for benign biliary obstruction depends on the clinical scenario, availability, and specific patient factors, the most common cause being a stone in the biliary system. Non-invasive methods like ultrasound and MRCP are preferred for initial evaluation, while invasive techniques like ERCP and PTC are reserved for more complex cases requiring therapeutic intervention [4].

2.2.1 Non-invasive imaging methods

2.2.1.1 Ultrasound

Ultrasound is often the first-line imaging modality due to its high specificity for cholelithiasis (**Figure 1**) and choledocholithiasis (bile duct stones) (**Figure 2**) and its ability to accurately identify the level and cause of biliary obstruction in most cases. Its advantages are cost-effectiveness, wide availability, and harmlessness [5].

2.2.1.2 Magnetic resonance cholangiopancreatography (MRCP)

MRCP (**Figure 3**) provides high-quality images of the biliary tree and is excellent for identifying the presence and level of biliary obstruction. Advanced techniques such as 3D gradient-echo (GRE) sequence in MRCP can help distinguish between benign and malignant strictures by showing changes in the bile duct wall and lumen [6].

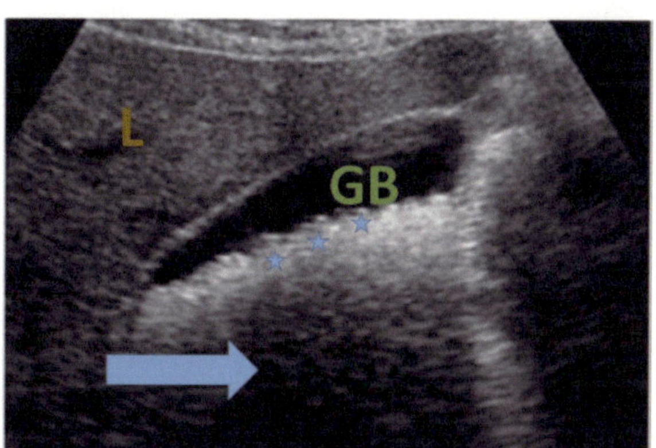

Figure 1.
Ultrasound image of cholelithiasis. L—liver, GB—gall bladder, asterixes—gall stones, blue arrow—acoustic or posterior shadowing.

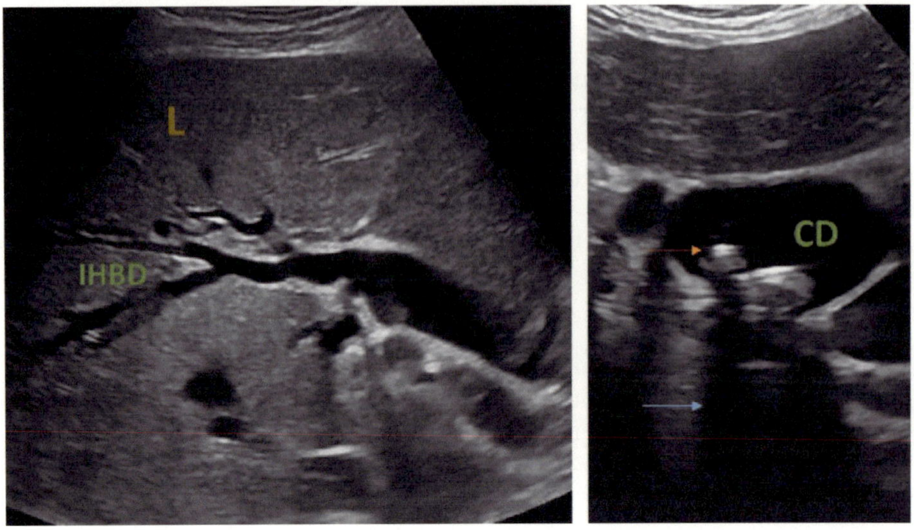

Figure 2.
Ultrasound image of choledocholithiasis. L—liver, IHBD—intrahepatic bile ducts, CD—choledochal duct, orange arrow—stone in choledochal duct, blue arrow—acoustic or posterior shadowing.

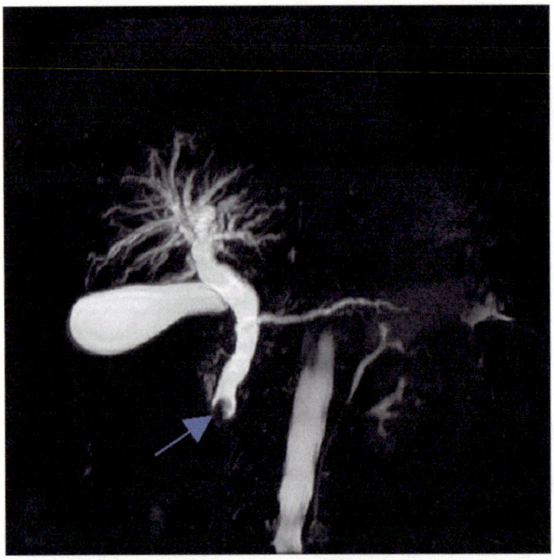

Figure 3.
Hypointense stone (blue arrow) in distal part of dilated choledochal duct-gall bladder and dilated gall ducts are hyperintense, stone has no signal intensity (MRCP, reconstructed).

2.2.1.3 Computed tomography (CT)

Multidetector CT (MDCT—**Figure 4**) offers detailed evaluation of the biliary tree with faster scanning and improved three-dimensional assessment, making it useful for diagnosing benign biliary strictures [7]. CT cholangiography provides high-resolution images and can be used to identify biliary pathology [8].

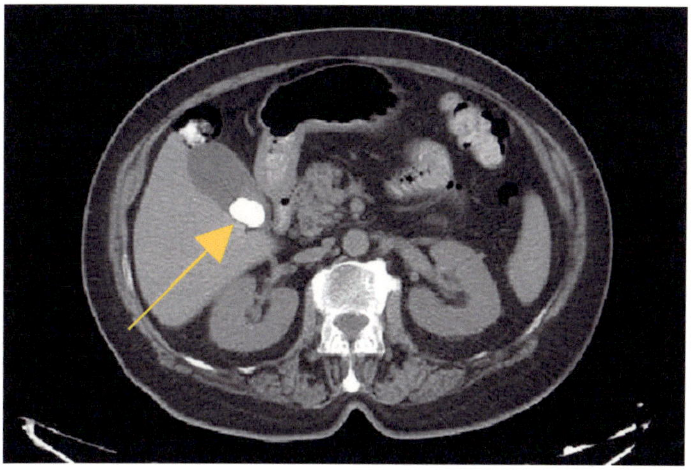

Figure 4.
Hyperdense X-ray positive stone (yellow arrow) in the gall bladder (native CT, axial view).

2.2.2 Invasive imaging methods

2.2.2.1 Endoscopic retrograde cholangiopancreatography (ERCP)

ERCP is the invasive diagnostic procedure of choice (**Figure 5**), allowing both localization of strictures and therapeutic interventions such as stenting. Combination with endoscopic ultrasound (EUS) can be used alongside ERCP for better visualization and tissue sampling [7].

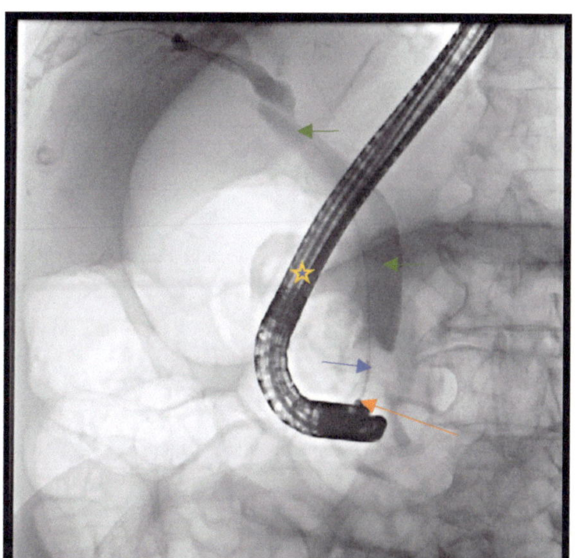

Figure 5.
ERCP—endoscopic device (asterix) is inside the duodenum, catheter (blue arrow) is placed through the papilla of Vateri (orange arrow), and iodine contrast media is injected into biliary tree (green arrows).

2.2.2.2 Percutaneous transhepatic cholangiography (PTC)

PTC is the alternative approach used for patients who are not candidates for ERCP, providing diagnostic evaluation and therapeutic options such as biliary drainage and stenting [9].

A summary of imaging modalities used in cases of benign biliary obstruction is shown in **Table 2**.

2.3 Biliary malignancies

To differentiate between benign and malignant biliary neoplasms on imaging, several key features and imaging modalities can be utilized. Here on **Table 3** are the primary features for benign and malignant lesions:

Initial evaluation: Ultrasound is often the first imaging modality used due to its high spatial resolution and ability to differentiate fluid-filled structures from soft tissues and especially to exclude biliary stones [10].

CT is useful for detecting and staging biliary malignancies, including cholangiocarcinoma (**Figure 6**) and gallbladder cancer. Contrast-enhanced CT provides detailed images of the biliary tract and can help identify the extent of disease [11].

MRI, combined with magnetic resonance cholangiopancreatography (MRCP) and magnetic resonance angiography, is essential for diagnosing and staging biliary

Modality	Type	Advantages	Limitations
US	Non-invasive	Cost-effective, widely available, high spec. For stones	Operator-dependent, limited by patient habitus
MRCP	Non-invasive	High-quality images, detailed biliary tree visualization	Expensive, slow, less available
CT	Non-invasive	Detailed 3D assessment, fast	Radiation exposure, less specific than MRI
ERCP	Invasive	Diagnostic and therapeutic, high accuracy	Risk of complication, requires sedation
PTC	Invasive	Useful for non-ERCP, diagnostic, and therapeutic	Risk of complication, invasive

Table 2.
Different imaging modalities used for liver and biliary tree—main advantages and disadvantages.

Feature	Benign	Malignant
Shape	Smooth, round	Lobulated, spiculated
Margins	Regular	Irregular
Signal intensity MRI	T1 homogenous, symmetric	T2 heterogeneous, asymmetric
DWI signal	Isointense	Hyperintense
Wall thickness	< 3 mm	> 3 mm
Length of stricture	Short	Long
Hyperenhancement (contrast techniques)	Absent	Present

Table 3.
Benign and malignant features of neoplasm.

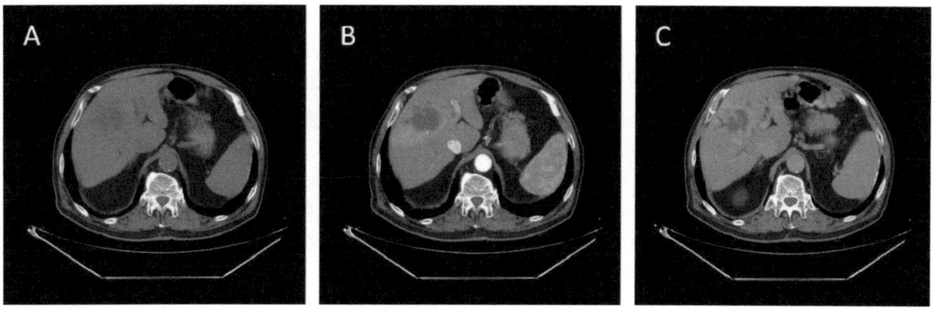

Figure 6.
Example of mass-forming, intrahepatic cholangiocarcinoma on computed tomography scan—different contrast phases-native scan without iodine contrast media (A), arterial phase (B), and portal or parenchymal phase (C) (CECT, axial view).

tumors. Diffusion-weighted imaging is useful for detecting nodal disease and peritoneal seeding [12].

PET/CT is particularly valuable for identifying distant metastases that may not be detected by other imaging modalities [12]. PET/CT findings can significantly alter the management plan by revealing unsuspected metastases [13].

Important imaging findings to take into consideration when reporting biliary malignancies are about the morphology and T-stage of primary tumor, M- and N-stage, and the presence of biliary obstruction, leading to cholestasis and the need of invasive procedures on the biliary tract (**Table 4**).

Primary tumor characteristics: masses and wall thickening—irregular thickening of the gallbladder or cyst wall, masses, and papillary nodules are indicative of malignancy. Marked enhancement after contrast administration can suggest malignancy.

Metastatic disease: PET/CT excels in identifying distant metastases, which are critical for staging and treatment planning [14]. Detection of regional lymph node metastases is crucial, though PET/CT may be less effective for this compared to distant metastases [13].

Biliary obstruction: Differentiating benign from malignant strictures is essential, with imaging playing a key role in defining the extent and guiding biopsy [15].

Role of interventional radiology is a diagnostic and therapeutic tool. Percutaneous drainage is used for managing biliary obstruction or leaks, either as a prelude to surgery or as palliative care. Biopsy and stent placement—techniques such as percutaneous transhepatic cholangiography (PTC) and endoscopic retrograde cholangiopancreatography (ERCP) are used for obtaining tissue samples and placing stents.

Imaging modality	Key uses	Strength
US	Initial evaluation, detection of obstruction, and stones	Real-time study, non-invasive
CT	Staging, detection of primary tumor	Detailed imaging, useful for surgical planning
MRI/MRCP	Comprehensive diagnosis and staging	Detailed soft tissue contrast
PET CT	N and M staging	Impact on management

Table 4.
Main uses of different imaging modalities for liver and biliary tree.

Special focus is set on magnetic resonance imaging (MRI) and magnetic resonance cholangiopancreatography (MRCP) as highly effective in differentiating benign from malignant biliary strictures. Malignant strictures often show irregular, asymmetric, and long-segment narrowing, while benign strictures typically present with regular, symmetric, and short-segment narrowing [16].

Contrast-enhanced MRI (CE-MRI) combined with MRCP can improve diagnostic accuracy. Malignant strictures are characterized by hyperenhancement relative to liver parenchyma, wall thickness > 3 mm, length > 12 mm, indistinct outer margins, luminal irregularity, and asymmetry (**Figure** 7).

Diffusion-weighted imaging (DWI) can further enhance the differentiation. Malignant lesions often appear hyperintense on high b-value DWI (b = 800 s/mm^2), which help distinguish them from benign lesions [17].

Combining CE-MRI, MRCP, and DWI significantly improves diagnostic accuracy. For instance, using three or more criteria from CE-MRI and MRCP can identify 100% of malignant strictures and 87% of benign strictures. MRCP alone has shown high diagnostic accuracy (93.3%) in differentiating benign from malignant biliary obstructions [18].

Direct cholangiography with tissue sampling remains the gold standard for definitive diagnosis. Combining multiple sampling techniques (e.g., forceps biopsy and brush cytology) can improve sensitivity [15].

2.4 Imaging after cholecystectomy

Understanding which are the common post-cholecystectomy complications can improve radiological assessment and early detection of these complications.

a. Biliary complications:

- Bile leaks
- Biloma[1]

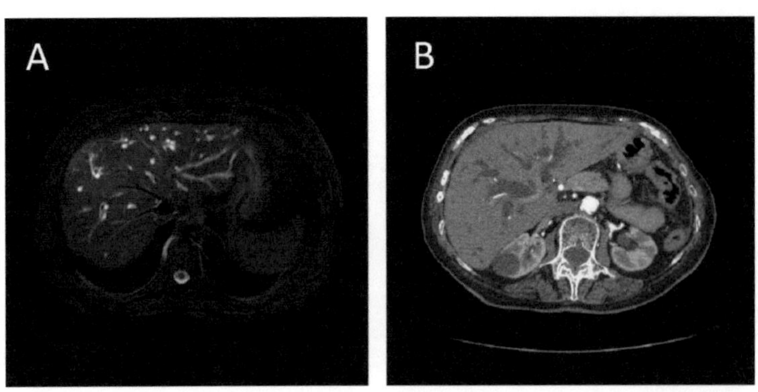

Figure 7.
Case of tumor of Klatskin-intraductal cholangiocarcinoma—no true mass-forming lesion is visible, but dilated ducts—hyperintense on T2 weighted sequence (A) and hypodense on computed tomography (B).

[1] *Biloma*, **Figure 8**, an encapsulated collection of bile outside the biliary tree, can result from traumatic, iatrogenic, or spontaneous causes. Imaging plays a crucial role in diagnosing and managing bilomas due to their often nonspecific clinical presentation.

- Biliary strictures

b. Stone-related complications:

- Retained/dropped stones
- Recurrent stones

c. Vascular complications:

- Hemorrhage and pseudoaneurysms

d. Infectious complications:

- Abscesses and infections

Imaging is indispensable in the postoperative evaluation of cholecystectomy patients. The choice of modality depends on the suspected complication and the clinical scenario. US and CT are commonly used first-line modalities, while MRCP and EUS offer detailed visualization for complex cases. Understanding the strengths and applications of each imaging technique is crucial for effective diagnosis and management of post-cholecystectomy complications [19].

2.4.1 Ultrasound (US)

Ultrasound (US) is the first-line modality: often used initially due to its availability and non-invasive nature [20], effective for detecting biliary dilatation, fluid collections, and gallstones.

2.4.2 Computed tomography (CT)

Computed tomography (CT) is widely used for comprehensive assessment of the postoperative abdomen, identifying complications such as abscesses, hematomas, and bile leaks. CT angiography may be helpful for many vascular complications and postoperative bleeding of unknown origin [21].

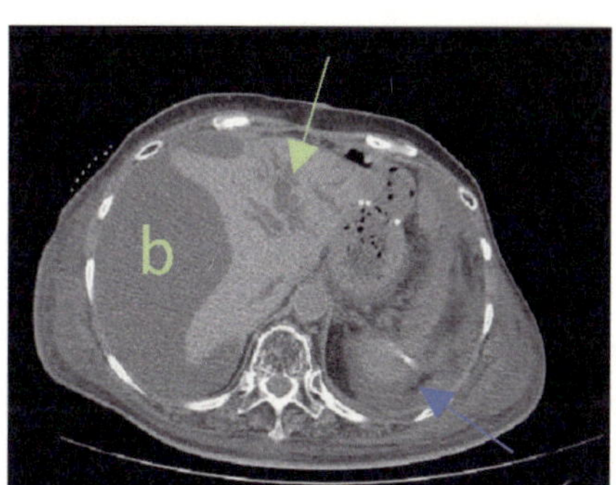

Figure 8.
Case of biloma-hypodense biloma (b) compressing the liver tissue, and dilated intrahepatic biliary ducts (green arrow) plus ascites (blue arrow) (contrast-enhanced computed tomography, axial view).

2.4.3 Magnetic resonance imaging (MRI) and magnetic resonance cholangiopancreatography

Magnetic resonance imaging (MRI) and magnetic resonance cholangiopancreatography is superior for detailed visualization of the biliary tree, identifying bile duct injuries, strictures, and retained stones. Gadoxetic acid-enhanced MRCP provides both anatomical and functional assessments of the biliary tract [22].

2.4.4 Endoscopic ultrasound (EUS)

Endoscopic ultrasound (EUS) is particularly useful for diagnosing stones in the cystic duct stump or gallbladder remnant, which may be missed by other modalities [23].

2.4.5 Scintigraphy

Scintigraphy is effective for diagnosing bile leaks, often used when other modalities are inconclusive.

Typical features of bilomas are well-defined fluid collections on imaging studies. Ultrasound may show an anechoic or hypoechoic area, while CT and MRI can provide more detailed anatomical information [24]. Imaging can also help identify complications such as infection, which may present as septations or increased fluid density. Management of biloma includes percutaneous drainage, often guided by ultrasound or CT, and follow-up imaging: regular imaging follow-up is essential to ensure resolution and detect any recurrence.

2.5 Imaging after biliary-enteric anastomosis

Biliary-enteric anastomosis (BEA) is a surgical procedure often performed for managing bile duct diseases, including benign and malignant conditions. However, this procedure can lead to several complications, which can be effectively identified and managed through various imaging techniques [25].

2.5.1 Common complications

a. *Bile leak*: This is an early complication that can be detected using imaging techniques such as MRI and CT scans.

b. *Biliary strictures*: These can occur both early and late post-surgery. Strictures are often identified through MR cholangiography (MRC) and can be managed with balloon dilatation and biliary drainage.

c. *Cholangitis*: This infection can be a result of bile stasis and is often detected through imaging showing bile duct dilation and fluid collections.

d. *Stones*: Formation of stones within the biliary system can be identified using MRI and CT scans.

2.5.1.1 Ultrasound

Useful for real-time assessment of bile duct dilation and fluid collections, though it may not provide detailed anatomical information.

2.5.1.2 Computed tomography (CT)

Widely available and provides detailed cross-sectional anatomy, useful for initial assessment.

2.5.1.3 Magnetic resonance imaging (MRI)

Particularly MR cholangiopancreatography (MRCP) is non-invasive and excels in visualizing bile ducts and detecting subtle changes in anastomosis integrity [26]. *T2-weighted MRCP* is effective for evaluating biliary-enteric anastomosis, though it lacks functional information (**Figure 9**).

2.5.1.4 MRCP

Contrast-enhanced MRCP provides both anatomical and functional information, which is useful for detecting strictures, stones, and bile leaks.

2.5.1.5 PTC

Percutaneous transhepatic cholangiography (PTC) is often used when endoscopic approaches are not feasible, such as in patients with Roux-en-Y anastomosis.

2.5.2 Management of complications

- *Balloon dilatation and biliary drainage:* Effective for treating benign biliary-enteric anastomosis strictures, with step-by-step balloon dilatation showing

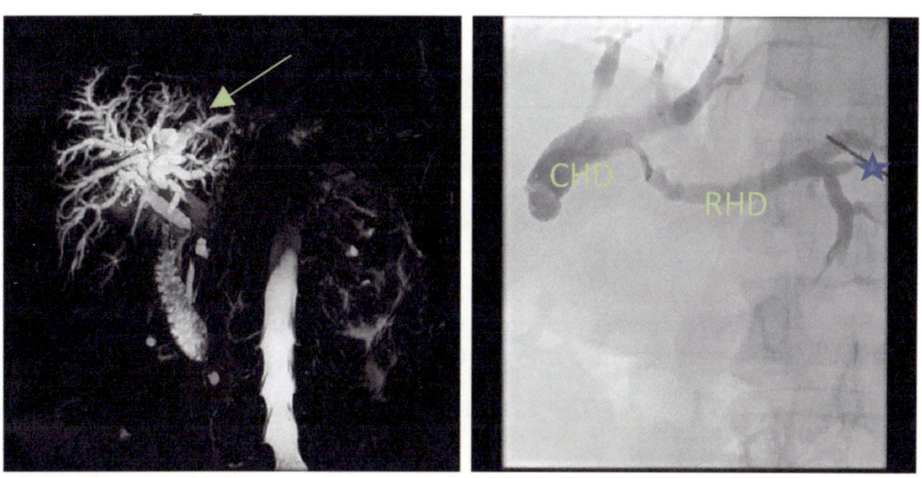

Figure 9.
Complicated case of Klatshin tumor and excessive dilation of biliary ducts—left picture MRCP and dilated ducts (green arrows), right picture PTC with radiopaque catheter (asterix) in biliary branch of right hepatic duct (RHD) and antegrade contrast administration into biliary tree (CHD—common hepatic duct).

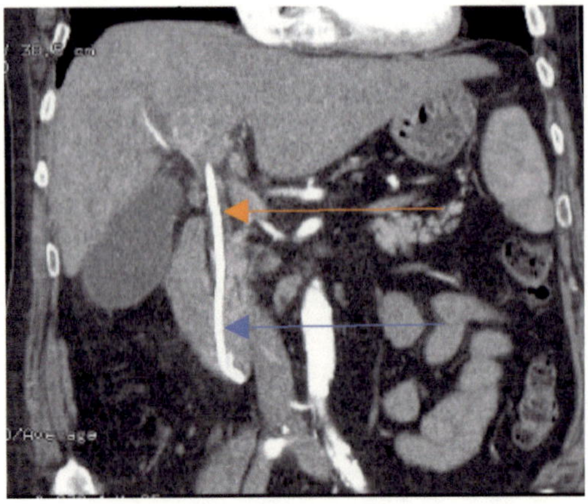

Figure 10.
Radiopaque biliary stent placement inside ductus choledochus (blue arrow) and ductus hepaticus communis (orange arrow) (contrast-enhanced computed tomography, coronal view).

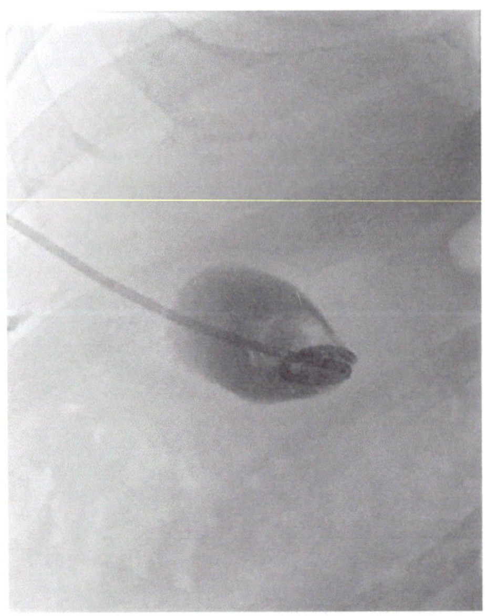

Figure 11.
Percutaneous transhepatic cholangiography (PTC) and catheter inside the gall bladder with radiopaque iodine contrast administration.

higher long-term patency rates. Stent placement into extrahepatic biliary ducts is another effective procedure (**Figure 10**).

- *Percutaneous interventions:* These include cholangiography and drainage, which are minimally invasive and effective for managing strictures and bile leaks (**Figure 11**).

- *Endoscopic retrograde cholangiopancreatography (ERCP):* Although challenging in BEA patients, it remains a valuable tool for diagnosis and treatment when feasible.

3. How to perform different imaging studies of biliary tree and gall bladder?

3.1 Ultrasound

3.1.1 Preparation

- Fasting: Ensure the patient has fasted for at least 6 hours to allow the gallbladder to be distended, which improves visualization.
- Positioning: The patient should lie in a supine position. Additional positions such as left lateral decubitus or upright may be used to improve visualization [27].

3.1.2 Technique

- Transducer selection: Use a lower frequency curvilinear transducer (3–5 MHz) for deeper structures.
- Initial survey: Begin with a general survey of the upper abdomen to locate the gallbladder and biliary tree [27].

3.1.3 Gallbladder evaluation

- Right subcostal approach: Place the transducer in the right subcostal region and use oblique sections to visualize the gallbladder [27].
- Longitudinal and transverse views: Obtain both longitudinal and transverse views to assess the gallbladder's size, wall thickness, and contents [27].
- Pathologies: Look for signs of cholecystitis, gallstones, polyps, and other abnormalities [28].

3.1.4 Biliary tree evaluation

- Common bile duct (CBD): Visualize the CBD by placing the transducer in the epigastric region and angling it toward the porta hepatis [27].
- Measurements: Measure the diameter of the CBD; a diameter greater than 6 mm may indicate dilation.
- Pathologies: Assess for biliary obstruction, stones, and tumors [29].

3.1.5 Key points

- Gallbladder: Evaluate for wall thickening, presence of stones, sludge, or masses.
- Biliary tree: Check for dilation, stones, and any masses within the bile ducts.
- Real-time monitoring: Use real-time ultrasound to guide interventions such as percutaneous biliary drainage if needed [30].

3.1.6 Common findings

- Cholelithiasis: Presence of echogenic foci with posterior acoustic shadowing within the gallbladder.
- Cholecystitis: Gallbladder wall thickening (>3 mm), pericholecystic fluid, and positive sonographic Murphy's sign.
- Biliary obstruction: Dilated intrahepatic bile ducts and CBD.

3.1.7 Advantages of ultrasound

- Non-invasive: No radiation exposure, making it safe for repeated use [30].
- Real-time imaging: Allows for dynamic assessment and immediate intervention if necessary.

3.1.8 Limitations

- Operator dependency: The quality of the examination is highly dependent on the skill and experience of the operator.
- Patient factors: Obesity and excessive bowel gas can limit the quality of the images [31].

3.2 Computed tomography

3.2.1 Preparation and protocol

- Ensure the patient is fasting for at least 4–6 hours before the scan to reduce the presence of bowel gas and improve visualization of the biliary tree and gall bladder [32].
- Contrast administration: Administer intravenous contrast material to enhance the visualization of vascular structures and biliary anatomy. In some cases, oral contrast may also be used [33].

3.2.2 Scanning technique

- Positioning: Position the patient supine on the CT table. Ensure the patient is comfortable to minimize movement during the scan.
- Scan phases: Utilize a triphasic examination technique, which includes:
- Non-contrast phase: Initial scan without contrast to identify calcifications and baseline anatomy.
- Arterial phase: Scan approximately 25–30 seconds after contrast injection to visualize arterial supply.
- Venous phase: Scan approximately 60–70 seconds after contrast injection to visualize venous structures and parenchymal enhancement.

- Delayed phase: Scan at 3–5 minutes post-contrast to assess for delayed enhancement patterns [34].

3.2.3 Image acquisition

- Thin collimation: Use thin collimation (e.g., 0.5–1 mm) to acquire high-resolution images. This allows for detailed multiplanar reconstructions and 3D imaging [35].

- Helical scanning: Employ helical scanning techniques to acquire volumetric data with sub-millimeter voxels, enabling detailed visualization of the biliary tree.

3.2.4 Post-processing

- Multiplanar reconstructions (MPR): Generate multiplanar reconstructions to visualize the biliary tree in different planes (axial, coronal, sagittal).

- Maximum intensity projection (MIP): Use MIP to highlight high-density structures such as bile ducts and vessels.

- Volume rendering: Apply volume rendering techniques to create 3D images that provide a comprehensive view of the biliary anatomy and any pathological lesions [35].

3.2.5 Diagnostic evaluation

- Assessment of pathology: Evaluate for biliary obstruction, gallstones, tumors, and anatomical variations. MDCT is particularly useful for staging gall bladder carcinoma and assessing the extent of disease spread.

- Vascular involvement: Assess the involvement of vascular structures to determine the resectability of tumors and plan surgical interventions.

3.2.6 Advantages of MDCT

- Speed and efficiency: MDCT allows for rapid scanning, reducing motion artifacts and improving image quality.

- Detailed visualization: Provides high-resolution images and detailed anatomical information, crucial for accurate diagnosis and treatment planning [36].

3.3 Magnet-resonance imaging

3.3.1 Preparation

- Ensure the patient fasts for at least 4–6 hours before the procedure to reduce the amount of fluid in the stomach and duodenum, which can interfere with imaging [36].

- Explain the procedure to the patient, including the need to remain still during the scan.

3.3.1.1 Equipment

- Use an MRI scanner with a high field strength (1.5 T or 3.0 T) to obtain high-resolution images.
- Ensure the availability of heavily T2-weighted sequences, which are essential for MRCP as they highlight static fluids like bile.

3.3.2 Imaging protocol

3.3.2.1 Positioning

- Position the patient supine on the MRI table.
- Use a phased-array body coil to enhance signal reception.

3.3.2.2 Sequences

- Heavily T2-weighted sequences: These sequences are crucial as they provide high contrast between the bile (which appears bright) and the surrounding tissues (which appear dark).
- 3D imaging: Utilize 3D sequences to allow for multiplanar reconstructions and detailed anatomical assessment.
- Single-shot fast spin-echo (SSFSE): This sequence is often used for rapid acquisition and to minimize motion artifacts [37].

3.3.2.3 Additional techniques

- Secretin stimulation: In some cases, secretin may be administered to enhance the visualization of the pancreatic ducts by increasing fluid secretion.
- Contrast-enhanced MRCP (CE-MRC): Although not always necessary, hepatobiliary-specific contrast agents can be used to improve the visualization of the biliary tree, especially in postoperative patients.

3.3.3 Procedure

3.3.3.1 Initial scans

- Begin with scout images to localize the biliary tree and gall bladder.
- Acquire heavily T2-weighted images in axial, coronal, and oblique planes to cover the entire biliary system.

3.3.3.2 Dynamic imaging

- If using secretin or contrast agents, perform dynamic imaging to capture the changes in the biliary and pancreatic ducts over time.

3.3.3.3 Post-processing

- Reconstruct 3D images to provide detailed views of the biliary anatomy and any pathological conditions.
- Use software tools to measure duct diameters and identify any strictures, stones, or other abnormalities.

3.3.4 Interpretation

- Qualitative assessment: Evaluate the images for the presence of biliary dilatation, stones, strictures, and anatomical variations.
- Quantitative biomarkers: Consider using quantitative measurements, such as duct diameters, to provide objective assessments.

3.3.5 Advantages of MRCP

- Non-invasive: No need for contrast agents or ionizing radiation.
- High sensitivity and specificity: Particularly effective for diagnosing biliary dilatation, choledocholithiasis, and anatomical variations.
- Comprehensive evaluation: Can be combined with conventional MRI to assess surrounding organs and tissues [38].

3.4 Endoscopic retrograde cholangiography

3.4.1 Patient selection

- Ensure appropriate patient selection and preparation, considering indications such as choledocholithiasis, biliary obstructions, and other biliary or pancreatic disorders.

3.4.2 Pre-procedural imaging

- Utilize imaging techniques like abdominal ultrasound or magnetic resonance cholangiopancreatography (MRCP) to confirm biliary tree dilatation and other relevant findings [39].

3.4.2.1 Procedure steps

1. Sedation and positioning: Administer sedation and position the patient appropriately, typically in the left lateral position.
2. Endoscope insertion: Insert a specialized side-viewing endoscope through the mouth, esophagus, and stomach into the duodenum.
3. Cannulation of the papilla of vater:
    - Locate the major duodenal papilla.

- Cannulate the papilla using a catheter or cannula.

4. Contrast injection:

    - Inject iodinated contrast material through the catheter to opacify the biliary and pancreatic ducts.
    - Use fluoroscopy to visualize the ducts and identify any abnormalities such as stones, strictures, or tumors.

5. Therapeutic interventions:

    - Stone extraction: Use tools like baskets or balloons to remove bile duct stones.
    - Stent placement: Insert stents to relieve obstructions caused by strictures or tumors.
    - Sphincterotomy: Perform a sphincterotomy if necessary to facilitate stone removal or stent placement [40].

3.4.2.2 Post-procedure care

- Fluoroscopic assessment: Conduct a post-procedural fluoroscopy study with contrast injection to ensure the effectiveness of the therapeutic interventions.
- Monitoring: Monitor the patient for potential complications such as pancreatitis, cholangitis, hemorrhage, and perforations [38].
- Follow-up: Schedule follow-up appointments to assess the patient's recovery and the success of the procedure.

3.4.2.3 Complications and management

- Common complications: Be aware of complications like post-ERCP pancreatitis, bleeding, and perforations. Early diagnosis and intervention are crucial for managing these complications.
- Management of complications: In cases of complications, consider conservative management, surgical intervention, or additional imaging as needed [41].

3.4.2.4 Advanced techniques

- Endoscopic ultrasound (EUS): Utilize EUS for additional diagnostic and therapeutic interventions, especially in complex cases or when ERCP fails [42].
- Peroral cholangioscopy (POC): Employ POC for high-definition imaging and targeted biopsies, enhancing the diagnostic accuracy and treatment outcomes [43].

3.5 Percutaneous transhepatic cholangiography

Overview: Percutaneous transhepatic cholangiography (PTC) is a diagnostic and therapeutic procedure used to visualize and treat conditions of the biliary tree and gall bladder. It involves the insertion of a needle through the skin and liver parenchyma into the intrahepatic bile ducts, followed by the injection of a contrast agent to display the biliary system.

3.5.1 Steps to perform PTC

1. Patient preparation:

    - Ensure the patient is appropriately sedated and positioned, typically in a supine position.

    - Perform a pre-procedural ultrasound to identify the biliary ducts and plan the needle insertion path.

2. Needle insertion:

    - Use a Chiba needle to puncture the skin and liver parenchyma under ultrasound or fluoroscopic guidance.

    - Aim for the intrahepatic bile ducts, ensuring to avoid vascular structures to minimize the risk of bleeding.

3. Contrast injection:

    - Once the needle is correctly positioned within the bile duct, inject a contrast agent to opacify the biliary tree.

    - Obtain fluoroscopic images to visualize the biliary anatomy and identify any obstructions or pathological changes.

4. Therapeutic interventions:

    - Depending on the findings, therapeutic interventions such as biliary drainage, stent placement, or stone extraction may be performed.

    - For biliary drainage, insert a catheter to decompress the biliary system, which can be external or internal-external.

- For stone extraction, use tools like lithotripsy devices, stone retrieval baskets, or mechanical fragmentation techniques [44].

3.5.2 Complications

- Minor complications include transient fever and minor bleeding.

- Severe complications can include significant bleeding, bile leaks, and infection [45].

3.5.3 Management

- Monitor the patient closely post-procedure for signs of complications.

- In case of bleeding, perform hepatic arteriography and embolization if necessary.
- Treat infections with appropriate antibiotics and supportive care.

3.5.4 Percutaneous transhepatic gallbladder drainage

- Indicated for patients with acute cholecystitis who are not candidates for early laparoscopic cholecystectomy.
- Involves the insertion of a drainage catheter into the gall bladder under imaging guidance.
- Can be combined with cholangiography to delineate biliary anatomy preoperatively.

4. Conclusion

Biliary imaging plays a pivotal role in the diagnosis and management of hepatobiliary diseases, offering detailed visualization of anatomical and pathological features. Advances in imaging modalities and contrast-enhanced techniques have significantly enhanced diagnostic accuracy and guided therapeutic interventions. Continued innovation and integration of imaging findings with clinical data remain essential for optimizing patient outcomes.

Acknowledgements

The authors acknowledge the use of Scopus AI for language polishing of the manuscript.

Conflict of interest

The authors declare no conflict of interest.

Author details

Tsvetelina Teneva[1*] and Aleksandar Zlatarov[2]

1 Medical University "Prof. P. Stoyanov", Varna, Bulgaria

2 University Hospital "St Marina", Varna, Bulgaria

*Address all correspondence to: tenevaz@gmail.com

References

[1] Modha K. Clinical approach to patients with obstructive jaundice. Techniques in Vascular and Interventional Radiology. 2015;**18**(4):197-200

[2] Karki S, Joshi KS, Regmi S, Gurung RB, Malla B. Role of ultrasound as compared with ERCP in patient with obstructive jaundice. Kathmandu University Medical Journal (KUMJ). 2013;**11**(43):237-240

[3] Briggs CD, Peterson M. Investigation and management of obstructive jaundice. Surgery (Oxford). 2007;**25**(2):74-80

[4] Fang A, Kim IK, Ukeh I, Etezadi V, Kim HS. Percutaneous management of benign biliary strictures. Seminars in Interventional Radiology. 2021;**38**(3):291-299

[5] Ghimire R, Lohani B, Pradhan S. Accuracy of ultrasonography in evaluation of level and cause of biliary obstruction: A prospective study. Kathmandu University Medical Journal (KUMJ). 2005;**3**(1):17-21

[6] Taheri A, Rostamzadeh A, Gharib A, Fatehi D. Efficacy of multidetector-row computed tomography as a practical tool in comparison to invasive procedures for visualization of the biliary obstruction. Acta Informatica Medica. 2016;**24**(4):257-260

[7] Fidelman N. Benign biliary strictures: Diagnostic evaluation and approaches to percutaneous treatment. Techniques in Vascular and Interventional Radiology. 2015;**18**(4):210-217

[8] Bill JG, Mullady DK. Stenting for benign and malignant biliary strictures. Gastrointestinal Endoscopy Clinics of North America. 2019;**29**(2):215-235

[9] Feldman MK, Coppa CP. Noninvasive imaging of the biliary tree for the interventional radiologist. Techniques in Vascular and Interventional Radiology. 2015;**18**(4):184-196

[10] Foley WD, Quiroz FA. The role of sonography in imaging of the biliary tract. Ultrasound Quarterly. 2007;**23**(2):123-135

[11] Matos C, Serrao E, Bali MA. Magnetic resonance imaging of biliary tumors. Magnetic Resonance Imaging Clinics of North America. 2010;**18**(3):477-496 x

[12] Petrowsky H, Wildbrett P, Husarik DB, Hany TF, Tam S, Jochum W, et al. Impact of integrated positron emission tomography and computed tomography on staging and management of gallbladder cancer and cholangiocarcinoma. Journal of Hepatology. 2006;**45**(1):43-50

[13] Girod BJ, Kandathil A. A review of F-18 fluorodeoxyglucose PET/CT in the evaluation and treatment of hepatobiliary tumors. The Quarterly Journal of Nuclear Medicine and Molecular Imaging : Official Publication of the Italian Association of Nuclear Medicine (AIMN) [and] the International Association of Radiopharmacology (IAR), [and] Section of the Society of Radiopharmaceutical Chemistry and Biology. 2024;**68**(4):245-258

[14] Shanbhogue AKP, Tirumani SH, Prasad SR, Fasih N, McInnes M. Benign biliary strictures: A current comprehensive clinical and imaging review. AJR. American Journal of Roentgenology. 2011;**197**(2):W295-W306

[15] Suthar M, Purohit S, Bhargav V, Goyal P. Role of MRCP in differentiation of benign and malignant causes of biliary obstruction. Journal of Clinical and Diagnostic Research : JCDR. 2015;**9**(11):TC08-TC12

[16] Lee NK, Kim S, Seo HI, Kim DU, Woo HY, Kim TU. Diffusion-weighted MR imaging for the differentiation of malignant from benign strictures in the periampullary region. European Radiology. 2013;**23**(5):1288-1296

[17] Sundaram KM, Morgan MA, Itani M, Thompson W. Imaging of benign biliary pathologies. Abdominal Radiology (New York). 2023;**48**(1):106-126

[18] Patel N, Jensen KK, Shaaban AM, Korngold E, Foster BR. Multimodality imaging of cholecystectomy complications. Radiographics : A Review Publication of the Radiological Society of North America, Inc. 2022;**42**(5):1303-1319

[19] Maddu K, Polireddy K, Hsu D, Hoff C. Do not get stumped: Multimodality imaging findings of early and late post-cholecystectomy complications. Emergency Radiology. 2023;**30**(3):351-362

[20] Tonolini M, Ierardi AM, Patella F, Carrafiello G. Early cross-sectional imaging following open and laparoscopic cholecystectomy: A primer for radiologists. Insights Into Imaging. 2018;**9**(6):925-941

[21] Gorsi U, Gupta P, Kalra N, Kang M, Singh R, Gupta R, et al. Multidetector computed tomography evaluation of post cholecystectomy complications: A tertiary care center experience. Tropical Gastroenterology : Official Journal of the Digestive Diseases Foundation. 2015;**36**(4):236-243

[22] Mohamadnejad M, Hashemi SJ, Zamani F, Baghai-Wadji M, Malekzadeh R, Eloubeidi MA. Utility of endoscopic ultrasound to diagnose remnant stones in symptomatic patients after cholecystectomy. Endoscopy. 2014;**46**(8):650-655

[23] Della Valle V, Eshja E, Bassi EM. Spontaneous biloma: A case report. Journal of Ultrasound. 2013;**18**(3):293-296

[24] Idriss AM, Tfeil Y, Baba JS, Abdallahi AM, Bezeid A. Non postoperative biloma in Mauritania: Case report and literature review. The Pan African Medical Journal. 2018;**31**:237

[25] Gawlik C, Carneval M. A review of the management of bile leaks. Cureus. 2021;**13**(5):e14937

[26] Boraschi P, Donati F. Biliary-enteric anastomoses: Spectrum of findings on Gd-EOB-DTPA-enhanced MR cholangiography. Abdominal Imaging. 2013;**38**(6):1351-1359

[27] Popescu A, Sporea I. Ultrasound examination of normal gall bladder and biliary system. Medical Ultrasonography. 2010;**12**(2):150-152

[28] Wills M, Harvey CJ, Kuzmich S, Afaq A, Cosgrove D. Ultrasound of the gall bladder and biliary tree: Part 2. British Journal of Hospital Medicine (London, England : 2005). 2014;**75**(6):318-324

[29] Segura Grau A, Joleini S, Díaz Rodríguez N, Segura Cabral JM. Ultrasound of gallbladder and bile duct. Semergen. 2016;**42**(1):25-30

[30] Müller T, Braden B. Ultrasound-guided interventions in the biliary system. Diagnostics (Basel, Switzerland). 2024;**14**(4):403

[31] Griffin S. Feline abdominal ultrasonography: What's normal? What's abnormal? The biliary tree. Journal of Feline Medicine and Surgery. 2019;**21**(5):429-441

[32] Lee JY. Multidetector-row CT of malignant biliary obstruction. The Korean Journal of Gastroenterology = Taehan Sohwagi Hakhoe chi. 2006;**48**(4):247-255

[33] Mohakud S, Sidhu S, Deep N, Naik S. Panorama of multidetector-row computed tomography findings of carcinoma gall bladder - A retrospective observational study. Journal of Cancer Research and Therapeutics. 2022;**18**(3):661-667

[34] Hashimoto M, Itoh K, Takeda K, Shibata T, Okada T, Okuno Y, et al. Evaluation of biliary abnormalities with 64-channel multidetector CT. Radiogr Rev Publ Radiol Soc N Am Inc. 2008;**28**(1):119-134

[35] Kim MJ, Choi JY, Chung YE. Evaluation of biliary malignancies using multidetector-row computed tomography. Journal of Computer Assisted Tomography. 2010;**34**(4):496-505

[36] Maccioni F, Martinelli M, Al Ansari N, Kagarmanova A, De Marco V, Zippi M, et al. Magnetic resonance cholangiography: Past, present and future: A review. European Review for Medical and Pharmacological Sciences. 2010;**14**(8):721-725

[37] Prabhakar PD, Prabhakar AM, Prabhakar HB, Sahani D. Magnetic resonance cholangiopancreatography of benign disorders of the biliary system. Magnetic Resonance Imaging Clinics of North America. 2010;**18**(3):497-514 xi

[38] Mousa HM, Hefny AF, Abu-Zidan FM. Life-threatening duodenal perforation complicating endoscopic retrograde cholangiopanceatography: A case series. International Journal of Surgery Case Reports. 2020;**66**:404-407

[39] Almuhaidb A, Olson D, Aadam AA. Advancements in endoscopic biliary interventions by gastroenterology. Seminars in Interventional Radiology. 2021;**38**(3):280-290

[40] Hormati A, Alemi F, Mohammadbeigi A, Sarkeshikian SS, Saeidi M. Prevalence of endoscopic retrograde cholangiopancreatography complications and amylase sensitivity for predicting pancreatitis in ERCP patients. Gastroenterology Nursing : The Official Journal of the Society of Gastroenterology Nurses and Associates. 2020;**43**(5):350-354

[41] Bang JY, Hawes R, Varadarajulu S. Endoscopic biliary drainage for malignant distal biliary obstruction: Which is better – Endoscopic retrograde cholangiopancreatography or endoscopic ultrasound? Digestive Endoscopy. 2022;**34**(2):317-324

[42] Pizzicannella M, Boskoski I, Perretta S. Peroral cholangioscopy: How technology and imaging have changed ERCP. Journal of Laparoendoscopic & Advanced Surgical Techniques. Part A. 2020;**30**(9):973-979

[43] Rousslang LK, Faruque O, Kozacek K, Meadows JM. Percutaneous transhepatic cholangioscopy and stone extraction in a patient with recurrent cholangitis following liver trauma. Journal of Clinical Imaging Science. 2021;**11**:11

[44] Widyaningtiyas I, Sarastika HY, Utama HW. Bleeding after percutaneous transhepatic biliary drainage due to arterial injury: A case study in patient with stable hemodynamic. Radiology Case Reports. 2022;**17**(12):4868-4873

[45] Yu B, Zhi X, Li Q, Xu B, Dong Z, Li T, et al. The efficacy and safety of preoperative cholangiography via percutaneous transhepatic gallbladder drainage (PTGBD) for difficult laparoscopic cholecystectomy (LC). Surgical Endoscopy. 2022;**36**(2):1355-1361

Chapter 4

Boon, Banes, and Cholecystectomy

Vania Myralda Giamour Marbun, Indah Jamtani, Karl Heinz Leonhardt Rowika and Nafilla Nesantya Sabatini

Abstract

Cholecystectomy is one of the most frequently performed surgical procedures worldwide, primarily indicated for the management of gallbladder conditions such as cholecystolithiasis and cholecystitis. While this procedure generally results in favorable clinical outcomes, it is not without potential complications, which can pose significant challenges for the patient and the surgeon. A comprehensive understanding of biliary anatomy is crucial to mitigate such risks. Furthermore, implementing bailout procedures illustrates surgeons' need to exhibit adaptability and humility while acknowledging their limitations to prioritize patient safety. This chapter explores these dual aspects and emphasizes the importance of understanding cholecystectomy's associated risks and benefits in improving patient care.

Keywords: cholecystectomy, critical view of safety, critical view of Strasberg, bile duct injury, laparoscopy cholecystectomy, double-window view, cystic duct, cystic artery, fundus down, top-down technique

1. Introduction

1.1 Historical glimpse of first cholecystectomy

> *"April 1882. Fresh, white sheets were brought down from the linen cupboard and laid over the kitchen table. A down pillow was placed under the head of the jaundiced 70-year-old woman; she was febrile, nauseated, crippled with abdominal and back pain, and clearly in extremis. Dr. William Steward Halsted carefully examined his patient, working his way to an inflamed mass on the right side of her abdomen just beneath the rib cage. The instruments he brought with him were boiled and dipped in carbolic acid. He rolled his coat sleeves above his wrists, washed his hands with green soap, dipped them in carbolic acid, and approached the patient, who was now breathing ether fumes and unaware of the impending surgery. With a scalpel in his bare hands, he cut through the tense skin and subcutaneous fat above the hot mass, then swiftly through rectus abdominus muscle and the peritoneum lining the abdomen, exposing the enlarged, pus-filled gallbladder. Halsted incised the inflamed organ, releasing a flood of purulent material and seven gallstones. Releasing the accumulation of pus and removing the gallstones effectively relieved the acute problem. William Stewart Halsted had successfully performed the first known operation to remove gallstones, and in the process had brought his mother back from the brink of death."*

Excerpt from the prologue of "Genius on The Edge: The Bizarre Double Life of Dr. William Stewart Halsted."

by Gerald Imber [1]

1.2 The history

The first cholecystectomy was performed by German surgeon Carl Johann August Langenbuch on a 42-year-old man on July 15, 1882. Before this, gallbladder surgeries were limited to stone removal, abscess drainage, or widening cholecystic fistulas [2]. Florentine pathologist Antonio Benivieni documented gallstones in 1420, noting a woman's death from abdominal pain, which raised awareness of biliary colic. Francis Glisson, named after the liver capsule, described his biliary colic as "from which there is no release except by death" in 1658 [3, 4].

The first gallstone surgery occurred in 1687 when Stalpert von der Wiel found gallstones in a patient with severe abdominal pain. However, the title of "father of gallbladder surgery" goes to Jean-Louis Petit, a Parisian surgeon who advocated removing gallstones and creating a biliary fistula for gallbladder abscesses in 1733, performing the surgery in 1743 [3]. In 1859, J.L. W Thudichum proposed a two-stage cholecystostomy, sewing the inflamed gallbladder to the abdominal wall in the first stage and later removing the stone through this stoma [4]. Gallstone surgery continued with the removal of stones and the creation of fistulas for some time. In 1867, John Stough Bobbs, a surgeon in Indianapolis, incidentally discovered gallbladder stones in a woman undergoing ovarian cyst surgery. He removed the stones, sutured the gallbladder, and left it in the abdomen. In 1878, Marion Simms coined the term cholecystostomy and was credited with designing, perfecting, and performing the first cholecystostomy [3, 4].

Carl Johann August Langenbuch first noted that relief from stone removal and cholecystostomy was temporary, stating, "They focus on the symptoms, not the cause." He studied gallbladder function and found that it wasn't essential for survival based on earlier experiments by Zambecarri in 1630 and Tenckhoff in 1667. Some colleagues believed the gallbladder aided stone formation. In July 1882, after 10 years of cadaver dissections and developing a removal technique, Dr. Langenbuch performed the first gallbladder removal cholecystectomy [3, 4]. Dr. Langenbuch performed cholecystectomies, endorsing the procedure for removing the gallbladder and addressing gallstone disease directly [2–4].

Langenbuch's open cholecystectomy was the gold standard for gallstone treatment until laparoscopic techniques emerged in the late nineteenth and early twentieth centuries [4, 5]. Philippe Mouret of Lyon is credited with the first laparoscopic cholecystectomy in 1987, although German surgeon Mühe attempted endoscopic gallbladder removal in 1985 using the galloscope, which had side optics and valves. Mühe later switched to a mini-laparotomy with a 2.5 cm incision. In 1987, Mouret's technique using four trocars, one for the laparoscope, became the standard. Dubois, from Paris, published the first report in May 1989, after learning from Mouret and performing successful tests before treating patients [5].

Today, the history of cholecystectomy shows steady improvement. This procedure evolved from Langenbuch's open surgery to today's advanced laparoscopic techniques, making it a safe option for millions globally. Ongoing advancements in surgical technology are expected to enhance the outcomes and safety of gallbladder removal.

DOI: http://dx.doi.org/10.5772/intechopen.1010679

2. The structure

2.1 The tree and its functions: Anatomy and physiology

The gallbladder is an organ located beneath liver segments IV and V. It measures approximately 7–10 cm long and 4 cm wide. It lies between the liver and peritoneum, lacks a capsule, and comprises three parts: a broad fundus, a tapering body leading to the infundibulum, and a narrow neck connecting to the cystic duct. Hartmann's pouch, an occasional fold at the neck-cystic duct junction, is a common site for gallstone impaction and mucocele formation. The cystic duct features spiral folds of mucosa, called the valves of Heister, which support duct patency and assist in controlling bile movement [6, 7].

Blood supply to the gallbladder primarily comes from the cystic artery, typically a branch of the right hepatic artery. The common bile duct is vascularized by branches from the proper hepatic, right gastric, and gastroduodenal arteries. Variations in cystic artery and gallbladder anatomy will be discussed separately.

Functionally, the gallbladder stores bile during fasting and releases it during meals. Hepatocytes produce bile, which flows through canaliculi between liver cells. Bile composition includes bile salts, cholesterol, and phospholipids, with most of the water drawn in osmotically. Concentration within the gallbladder increases bile potency five to tenfold, lessening the volume for storage. As bile travels through the ducts, bicarbonate, water, glucose, and amino acids are secreted or reabsorbed, modifying its composition [8].

Bile transport varies between the fasting and feeding phases. In fasting, high hepatic pressure and a relaxed gallbladder allow bile to flow in, while the sphincter of Oddi remains closed. During digestion, cholecystokinin (CCK) and acetylcholine trigger sphincter relaxation and gallbladder contraction, releasing bile into the duodenum to aid in fat digestion and absorption (**Figure 1**) [8, 9].

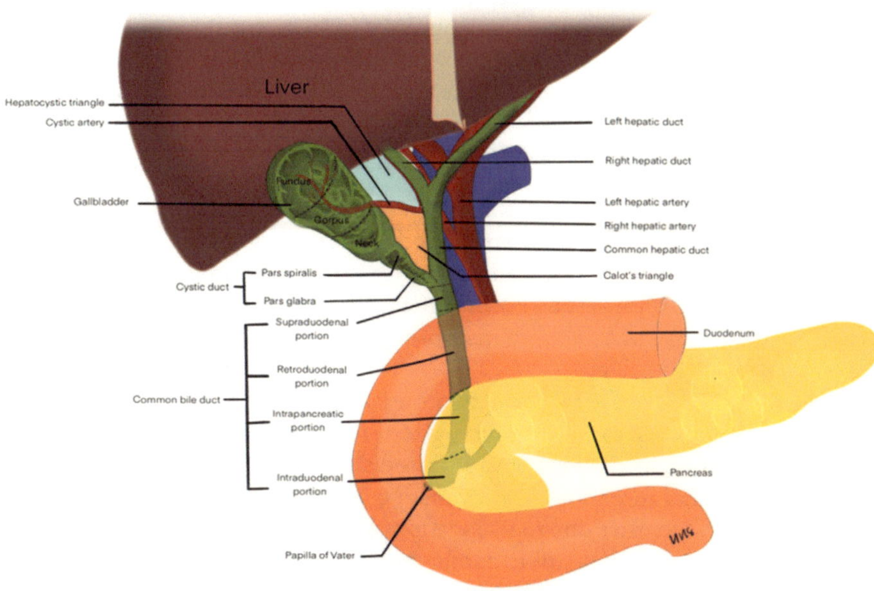

Figure 1.
Anatomy of the biliary system.

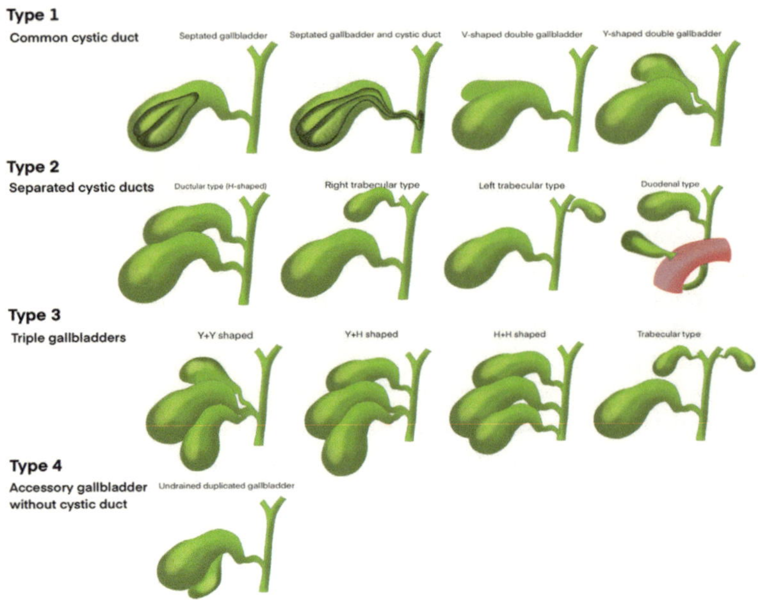

Figure 2.
Variations of multiple gallbladders according to Harlaftis classification [11], including all subtypes of variation.

2.2 From pear-shaped to peculiar: Variations of gallbladders

A deviation from normal anatomical development is the cause of all gallbladder variations. The gallbladder varies in size and shape. The fundus may be quite movable and extended. On rare occasions, the fundus, also known as a Phrygian cap, curls over the corpus and could be mistaken for a septum on ultrasonography [10].

Boyden and Harlaftis et al. categorized gallbladder variations [11], who described the double gallbladder and its varied morphology in 1926. No signs or symptoms are connected to having two gallbladders. It has not been established that a duplicate gallbladder has a higher disease prevalence than a single gallbladder (**Figure 2**).

2.3 Cystic ducts and detours: Variations of cystic ducts

The cystic duct connects the gallbladder to the extrahepatic bile duct, marking the junction between the common hepatic and common bile ducts. The cystic duct typically measures 2–4 cm and contains concentric mucosal folds called the valves of Heister. In most cases, it joins the extrahepatic bile duct midway between the porta hepatis and ampulla of Vater, though insertion points can vary from high near the porta to low near the ampulla.

Congenital variations of cystic duct anatomy are common. Around 75% insert at the middle third of the extrahepatic duct, often from a right lateral approach. Other patterns include spiral, low lateral with a shared sheath, proximal, and low medial insertions. Low medial insertion may be misdiagnosed on imaging (CT, MRI, or US) as a septated cystic structure due to its location and course through the pancreatic head. These insertions often result in a longer cystic duct remnant. While most bile duct anomalies are not clinically significant, accessory ducts, especially from the right lobe, can join near the cystic duct and increase the risk of accidental injury during cholecystectomy (**Figure 3**) [13].

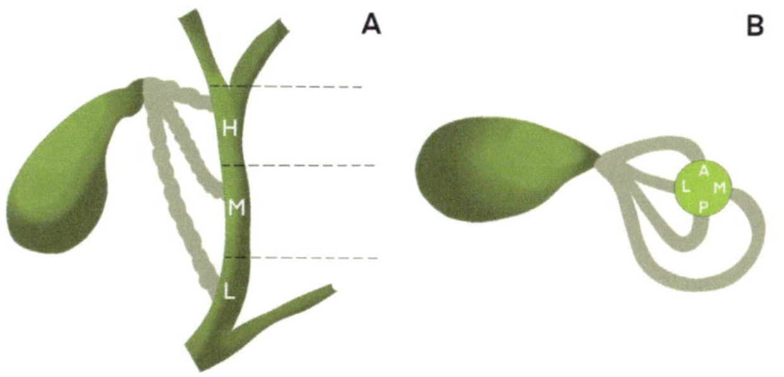

Figure 3.
[A] In coronal view, H (high), M (mid), and L (low) show the level of cystic duct insertion at the extrahepatic bile duct. [B] In axial view, L (lateral), A (anterior), M (medial), and P (posterior) show the point of insertion at the extrahepatic duct [12].

2.4 Variations of cystic artery

The cystic artery shows significant anatomical variability, which is critical to consider during cholecystectomy. According to a comprehensive systematic review and meta-analysis, the CA most commonly originates from the right hepatic artery (RHA) in 85.75% of cases. Other origins include the aberrant RHA (6.16%), proper hepatic artery (5.86%), gastroduodenal, left hepatic, common hepatic, and even the superior mesenteric and middle hepatic arteries. Most cystic arteries are single vessels (88.59%), but variations such as accessory arteries occur in about 8.59%, with rare cases of triplication or absence [14]. These variations can lead to complications if not properly identified and managed during surgery.

Most of the cystic artery is usually found inside the cystohepatic triangle (83.83%) and most often courses superomedial to the cystic duct. However, it may also lie anterior, posterior, or inferior to nearby ducts, such as the common hepatic and bile ducts. In 16.28% of cases, it lies outside the triangle, complicating surgical visualization [14].

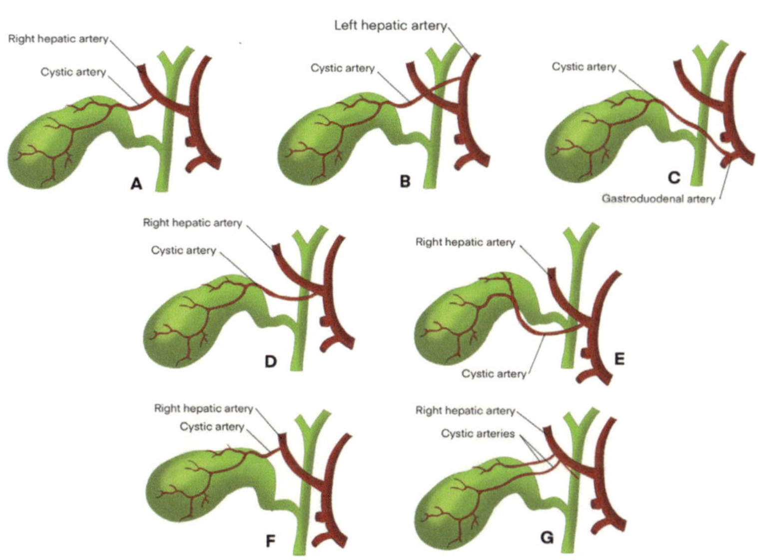

Figure 4.
Illustrations of commonly found variations of the cystic artery.

The length of the cystic artery may vary between 10 and 30 mm. This variability in origin, course, and morphology underlines the importance of meticulous dissection and identification during cholecystectomy to avoid iatrogenic injury (**Figure 4**) [14, 15].

3. How it all began: Open cholecystectomy

Cholecystectomy is a procedure to remove the gallbladder. It is one of the most common procedures in the United States, with more than 1.2 million procedures performed annually. Up until 1991, open cholecystectomy was the standard procedure for gallbladder removal, and it usually included an intraoperative cholangiogram. The length of stay ranges from 2 to 6 days [16].

Nowadays, the laparoscopic approach is favored over the open approach. However, the laparoscopic approach is associated with a higher incidence of bile duct injury, the injury increases by 3 to 10 times.

3.1 Operation technique

3.1.1 Position

The patient's position plays a crucial role in surgery. It has the advantage of helping the surgeon expose the gallbladder better in certain positions. First, the patient is secured at the operating table (fixing the patient's torso and hip is essential to prevent the patient from falling). The exposure can be enhanced by tilting the table to a level where the body is semi-erect. A slight tilt to the left side might come in handy to move the intestines to the left side of the body [17].

3.1.2 Operative preparation

The skin should be cleaned and the hair should be removed only with a clipper (only if necessary). Prophylactic antibiotics should also be given before the time of incision [17].

3.1.3 Incision and exposure

There are two main types of incision: the high midline incision and the oblique subcostal incision (Kocher incision). The midline incision gives the advantage of exposing other organs; hence, it is a preferable incision when other pathologies, such as hiatus hernia, duodenal ulcer, etc., are present. The subcostal incision has other advantages, such as good exposure, minimal early postoperative wound discomfort, and decreased risk of incisional hernia [17, 18].

The surgeon's preference determines which of the two incisions to use. The incision can be made with a scalpel or electrocautery [17, 18].

3.1.4 Details

After exposing the abdominal cavity, a self-retaining retractor can be used advantageously, allowing for the exploration of the liver and its surrounding organs for any sign of infection or pathology [17, 18].

Identify the gallbladder beneath the liver and use a clamp at its fundus to provide traction. Then, another clamp at the round ligament provides countertraction. Pull down the clamp holding the gallbladder toward the costal margin to present the undersurfaces of the liver and gallbladder [17, 18].

If a surgeon encounters an acutely inflamed and distended gallbladder, aspiration should be considered to prevent small stones from getting through the cystic and common duct. Adhesions are common around the gallbladder; some involve the duodenum or transverse colon and surrounding organs. The adhesions are divided using curved scissors or electrocautery until an avascular plane can be developed adjacent to the wall of the gallbladder. Afterward, it's possible to brush these adhesions with gauze sponges [17, 18].

After a clear vision of the gallbladder, the surrounding organs, such as the stomach or transverse colon, can be packed away using moist gauze pads and held with a retractor. This technique may give more space and a clearer view of the gallbladder [17, 18].

After clear exposure, the peritoneum is divided on the inferior aspect of the gallbladder and extends downward to the neck region. The dividing process could be achieved using an electrocautery or a long Metzenbaum dissecting scissors. Extend the incision downward toward the hepatoduodenal ligament, then clear the neck area of the gallbladder using blunt gauze dissection. After being exposed clearly, move the clamp from the fundus to the neck. Continue the dissection toward the cystic duct using blunt dissection until the cystic duct is identified. Using a long right-angle clamp to pass behind the cystic duct, slowly but surely with tremendous precision, the cystic duct is then isolated from the common duct and clamped (it would be wise to check one more time for any calculi in the common duct and the cystic duct before clamping the cystic duct). Also, isolate the cystic artery at any chance possible, especially when there are no signs of severe inflammation or adhesions. Never assume that a right-angle clamp could withhold both duct and artery included in one mass ligature [17, 18].

If necessary, an optional intraoperative cholangiography may be performed through the cystic duct after it has been divided. After the cholangiogram, the cystic duct is ligated with a transfixing suture or a ligature, making sure no common ducts or other vessels are included [17, 18].

After the cystic artery and duct are ligated, the surgeon may proceed by carefully separating the gallbladder from the bed liver, using electrocautery from the infundibulum toward the fundus until the gallbladder is detached from the liver completely [17, 18].

4. The pinnacle of gallbladder surgery: Laparoscopic cholecystectomy

4.1 Room setup

See **Figures 5** and **6**.

4.2 Operation technique

4.2.1 The preparation

The patient is administered with general anaesthesia and undergoes standard laparoscopic preparation [19–21]. A Foley catheter and nasogastric tube are inserted. An 11-mm trocar is positioned infraumbilical using the Hasson technique through a semilunar incision, serving as the access point for the laparoscopic camera. Carbon dioxide insufflation is initiated through the first trocar at a low to moderate flow rate, starting at 1.5 L/min, until the intra-abdominal pressure reaches 12 mmHg. The insufflation rate is then increased and maintained at a high rate of 7–10 L/min.

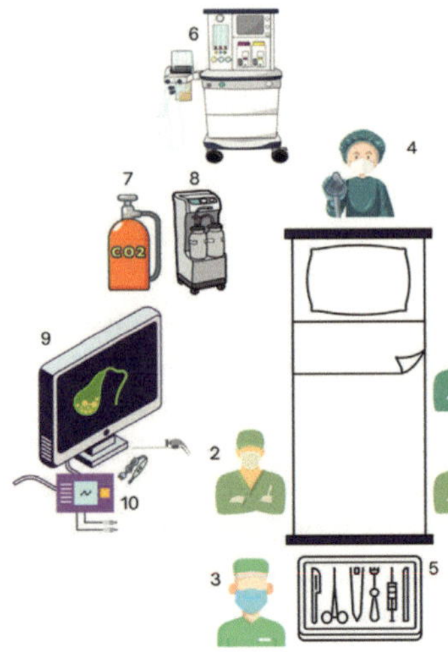

Figure 5.
(1) Surgeon; (2) Assistant; (3) Scrub nurse; (4) Anaesthesiologist; (5) Instrument table; (6) Anaesthesia machine; (7) Insufflator; (8) Suction machine; (9) Laparoscopic tower and monitor; (10) Cautery.

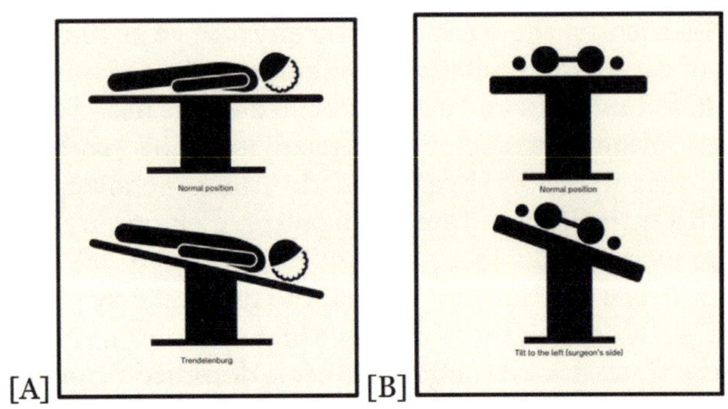

Figure 6.
Bed position in [A] sagittal view and [B] axial view.

The surgeon must visualize the underlying space to ensure that no bowel injury occurs during the trocar insertion. Subsequently, visual exploration is conducted to examine the internal organs in the upper abdomen.

A second 11-mm trocar is inserted beneath the xiphoid process to serve as the access point for the surgeon's right-hand instrument. A third 5-mm trocar is placed along the right midclavicular line for the operator's left-hand instruments, and an optional fourth trocar (4 mm) may be positioned near the right anterior axillary line (**Figure** 7).

4.2.2 The main act

The fundus is held and maneuvered cranially toward the right diaphragm or laterally toward the right abdominal wall until the Hartmann pouch is identified [19, 21]. This maneuver is performed to adequately expose the cystic duct, provided sufficient force is applied. Several safety landmarks may be used to identify the critical view of safety (CVS).

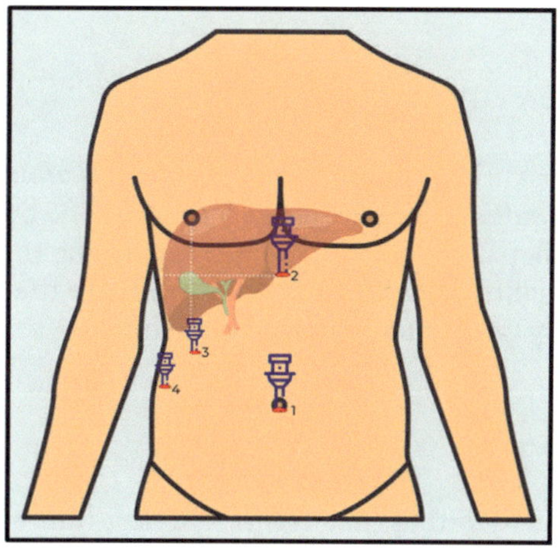

Figure 7.
Trocar placement in laparoscopic cholecystectomy. (1) Infraumbilical for camera port; (2) Epigastrium, below the edge of the liver; (3) Right quadrant, along the right midclavicular line; (4) Right quadrant, along the right anterior axillary line.

The dissection begins in parallel and perpendicular fashions at the anterior section using dissecting forceps, specifically Maryland forceps, along with monopolar devices or advanced ultrasonic or bipolar devices until the cystic duct and cystic artery are fully exposed.

The dissection may then progress to the left and right lateral aspects of the gallbladder, continuing until approximately one-third of the inferior gallbladder is detached from the cystic plate. When the critical view of safety (CVS) is obtained, a doublet-view or double window will become evident, displaying the cystic duct, cystic artery, and liver parenchyma as the vertical structures within the window.

The two vital structures must be ligated upon identification of the critical view of safety (CVS) to minimize the risk of bile duct injury. This ligation should be performed using polymer or titanium clips to ensure secure double ligation. Following ligation, the structures are prepared for division using scissors, specifically Metzenbaum or hook scissors, to ensure safe and precise dissection.

The gallbladder is detached from the cystic plate utilizing a monopolar L-hook or spatula electrocautery on the operator's right hand. This is accomplished by elevating the neck of the gallbladder with the left-hand instrument until the junction between the serosal surface and the cystic plate is fully exposed.

4.2.3 The closure

When the fundus is the only portion still attached to the liver bed, it is crucial to inspect for hemostasis and any potential bile leaks using the aspirator – irrigator [19, 21]. Once it is confirmed that the area is secure, the fundus is detached and subsequently placed into the endobag. The endobag is previously inserted through the subxiphoid trocar and then exits through the infra-umbilical port immediately after being loaded with the gallbladder specimen.

It is essential to refrain from retracting the endobag to prevent intra-abdominal tearing. Always ensure that the specimen and gallstone are removed first, followed by the endobag.

4.3 Safety landmark

4.3.1 Critical view of safety (CVS)

CVS is a method of identifying two critical structures, which are cystic duct and cystic artery, to achieve safe cholecystectomy. It can be done by (1) clearing fat and fibrous tissue from the hepatocystic triangle; (2) separating the lower one-third of the inferior part of the gallbladder from the liver to expose the cystic plate; and (3) identifying two and only two structures should be seen entering the gallbladder (**Figure 8**).

4.3.2 The sulcus of Rouviere

In 1957, Claude Coinaud, rather than Henri Rouviere himself, introduced the term "Rouviere sulcus. In 1924, Henri described the sulcus as "*Silon du processus caud*e," identifying it as a transverse groove between the caudate process and the right lobe of the liver [22–24]. This feature has since been acknowledged as a crucial safety landmark in laparoscopic cholecystectomy, although Henri was unaware of its clinical importance then. Thomas B. Hugh was the first to publish findings regarding the utilization of Rouviere's sulcus and to identify a safe dissection triangle associated with laparoscopic cholecystectomy (**Figure 9**) [22, 24, 25].

We can identify four types of Rouviere sulcus during laparoscopy: (1) open; (2) closed; (3) slit; and (4) scar. The importance of recognizing this structure lies in its precise indication of the plane of the common bile duct, which serves as a reference point for initiating dissection during laparoscopic procedures until the identification of the CVS. The cystic duct and cystic artery are located anteroposteriorly above the sulcus, while the common bile duct is beneath the sulcus.

4.3.3 B-safe

One of the main reasons for bile duct injury is anatomical misperception due to structure disorientation before dissection and ligation [26]. B-SAFE is an anatomical landmark used in laparoscopy cholecystectomy to help identify essential structures (**Figure 10** and **Table 1**) [26, 27].

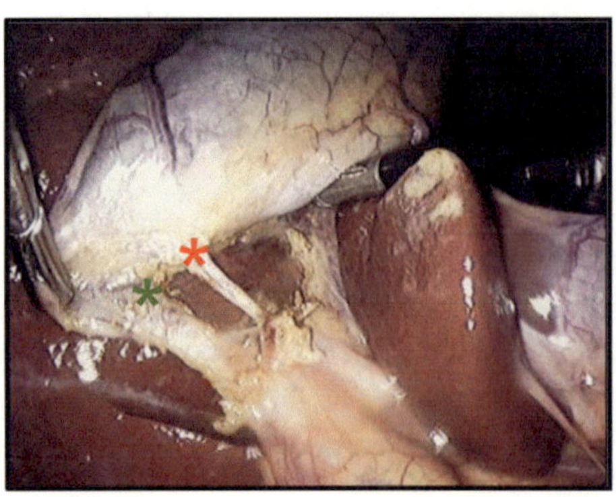

Figure 8.
Only two structures, the cystic duct (green asterisk) and the cystic artery (red asterisk), enter the gallbladder in the doublet view.

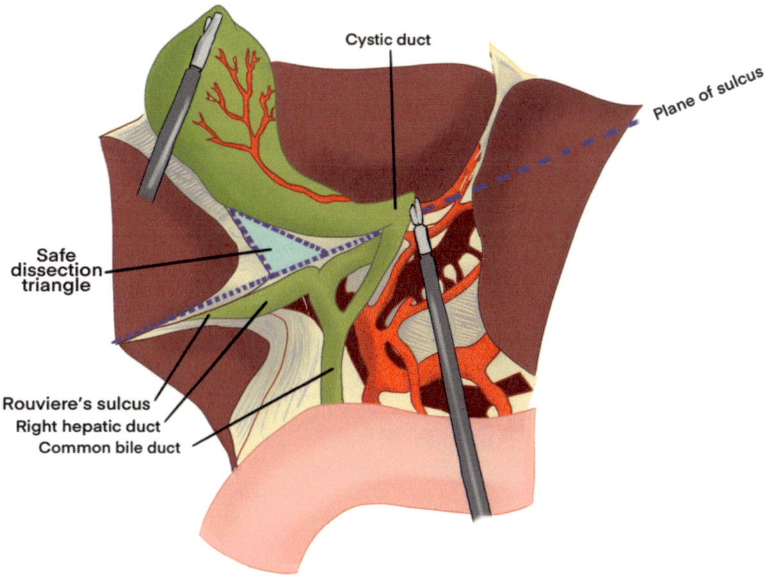

Figure 9.
The Sulcus of Rouviere along with the triangle of safe dissection. Remember to always start dissecting above the Rouviere's sulcus.

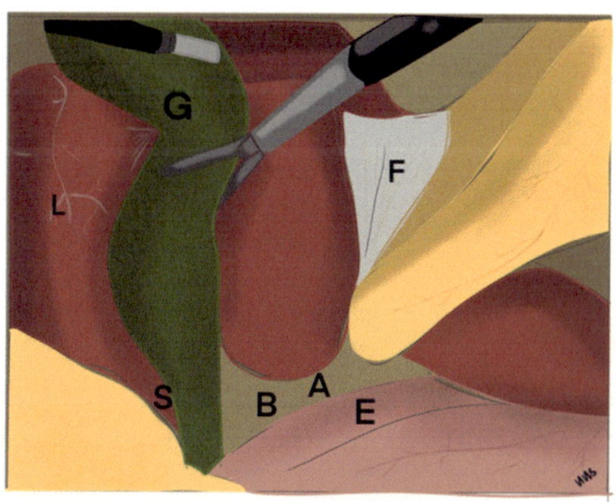

Figure 10.
Sketch of B-SAFE in laparoscopic cholecystectomy. L: liver; G: gallbladder; B: bile duct; S: sulcus of Rouviere; A: artery hepatica; F: falciform ligament; E: enteric viscera.

B	Bile duct, base of segment 4b
S	Sulcus of Rouviere
A	Artery hepatica
F	Fissura umbilicalis
E	Enteric viscera (duodenum)

Table 1.
Description of B-SAFE acronym.

4.3.4 R4U line

Another reference point deemed a "safe zone" for initiating dissection is the "R4U line." This line runs from the roof of the Rouviere sulcus to the base of segment 4b (quadrate lobe) and extends to the umbilical fissure. It serves as a foundation for two planes, the "A" plane and the "R" plane, which are typically perpendicular to one another, dividing the area into four surgical zones (**Figure 11**) [28].

The first zone is the antero-superior zone, which is identified as the only green zone, indicating it is the safest area for dissection. This zone includes the cystic duct

Line	Planes	"A" Plane			Zones
		Areas	Anterior	Posterior	
R4U	"R" Plane	Superior	Antero-superior	Postero-superior	
		Inferior	Antero-inferior	Postero-inferior	

[a]

Antero-superior	Postero-superior
Antero-inferior	Postero-inferior

[b]

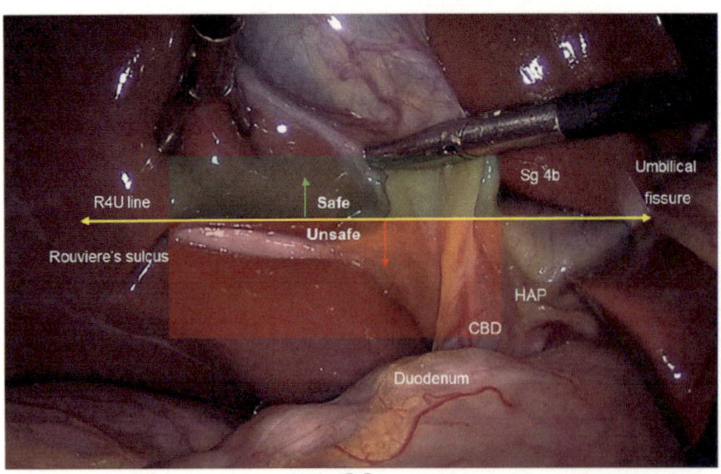

[c]

Figure 11.
[a] Concept of R4U planes dividing 4 zones: [b] Green zone (safe zone): antero-superior; orange zone (potentially dangerous zone): postero-superior, and red zone (most dangerous zone): both antero-inferior and postero-inferior. [c] The area above the R4U line is safe for starting dissection in laparoscopic cholecystectomy.

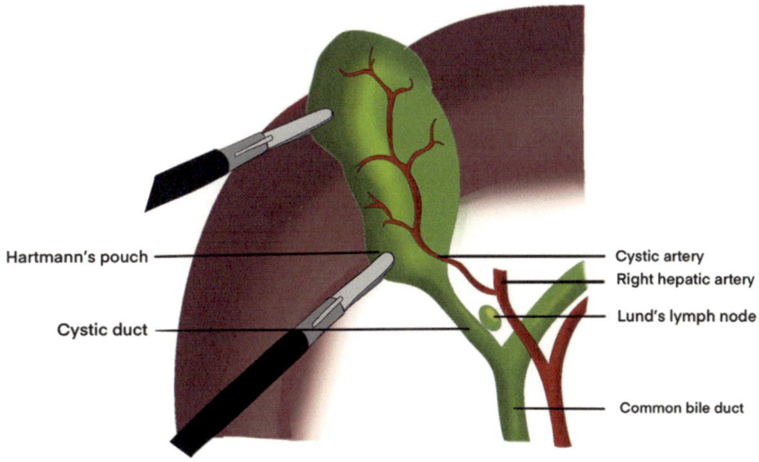

Figure 12.
Lund's lymph node.

and cystic artery. The postero-superior zone is classified as an orange zone or the potentially dangerous zone, where dissection must be done carefully to achieve CVS while being aware of key structures and not cutting too deeply. The other two inferior zones are referred to as the red zone, or the dangerous zone, where dissection is strongly prohibited.

4.3.5 Alternative landmarks

4.3.5.1 Lund's lymph node

This cystic lymph node can be used to identify the cystic artery because it is located at the exit of the cystic artery from the right branch of the proper hepatic artery (**Figure 12**) [29].

4.3.5.2 Injection of indocyanine green

The use of indocyanine green (ICG) aims to enhance the visualization of essential structures, such as the common bile duct and cystic duct, thereby minimizing the potential for anatomical misinterpretation and disorientation during surgery [30, 31]. Additionally, ICG can reduce the duration of surgical procedures, particularly in acute cases, by enabling quicker identification of these critical structures, thus lowering the risk of bile duct injuries. Two methods of administration are available: intravenously or directly into the gallbladder [32].

5. Rescue mission: The bailout procedure

5.1 Definition

Bailout originally came from the Latin word *baiulare,* meaning "to carry a load." Over time, its meaning evolved to "to rescue from a difficult situation." Currently, in laparoscopic cholecystectomy, the term is often used to describe intraoperative adjustments to procedural steps that are undertaken to facilitate the optimal removal of the gallbladder while ensuring the safety of the patient [33, 34].

5.2 Rules of engagement

Several intraoperative findings require a surgeon to do a time-out:

1. Severe fibrosis and scarring in Calot's triangle due to inflammation
2. Impacted gallstone in the confluence of the cystic, common hepatic, and common bile duct (included in the expanded classification of Mirizzi syndrome)
3. Anomalous bile duct
4. Extensive blood loss
5. Extensive and dense adhesion to surrounding organs and/or greater omentum
6. Severe fibrosis and scarring in gallbladder bed due to inflammation (includes sclero-atrophic gallbladder)
7. Extensive operative time

Based on the Delphi consensus among international laparoscopic surgeons, severe fibrosis in Calot's triangle has the highest response rate of 94.3% and is also identified as one of the most difficult intraoperative findings [35].

5.3 Subtotal cholecystectomy

In 2013, Henneman published a systematic review examining surgical approaches for complex gallbladder cases [36]. The review outlined four approaches:

a. Removing most of the anterior wall of the gallbladder while leaving part of the posterior wall attached to the liver.

b. Removing most of the anterior wall of the gallbladder while leaving part of the posterior wall attached to the liver, but with the remaining stump being closed.

c. Removing both the anterior and posterior walls at the level of Hartmann's pouch or the gallbladder neck, then closing the pouch.

d. Removing both the anterior and posterior walls at the level of Hartmann's pouch or the gallbladder neck without closing the pouch.

Strasberg also published an article about performing incomplete cholecystectomy in 2015 and clarified the difference between partial and subtotal cholecystectomy [37, 38]. Subtotal terminology is preferred to partial cholecystectomy in describing the extension of gallbladder removal (**Figure 13**).

In fenestrating cholecystectomy, the anterior portion of the gallbladder is excised until the lip is encountered, which serves as a protective barrier before accessing the hepatocystic triangle (referred to as the shield of McElmoyle). The gallstones are

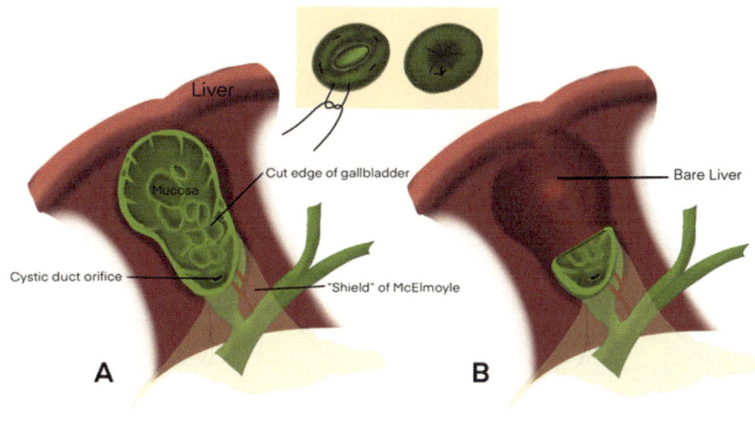

Figure 13.
In subtotal fenestrating cholecystectomy, we can either leave the posterior part of the gallbladder in situ [A] or excise the anterior and posterior parts of the gallbladder until the shield of McElmoyle is encountered [B].

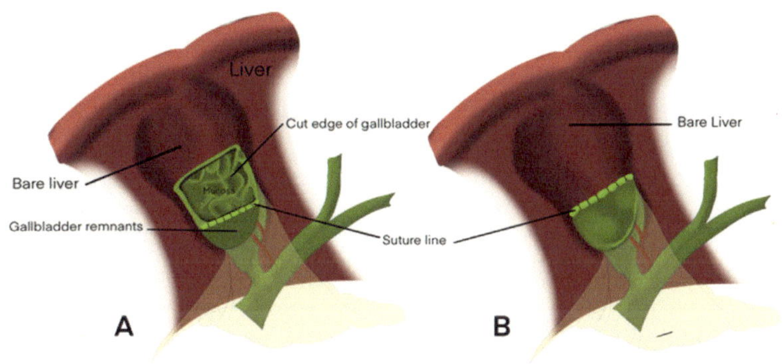

Figure 14.
In reconstituting cholecystectomy, the anterior portion of the gallbladder is excised, while the posterior segment may either be excised or left intact. The remaining part of the gallbladder is then sutured to facilitate reconstruction.

extracted, while the posterior part of the gallbladder that remains attached to the liver is left in place. The lip is subsequently closed using a purse-string technique from the inside, without closing the remnant part (**Figure 14**).

In reconstituting cholecystectomy, the anterior portion of the gallbladder is excised until the lip is encountered. The posterior part may be excised or left intact. After extracting the gallstones, the remaining anterior section is sutured to the posterior part to reconstruct the lumen. Care must be taken not to leave too much space to avoid the formation of new stones and the risk of post-cholecystectomy syndrome.

The distinction between these two types of subtotal cholecystectomy is not determined by the size of the remaining gallbladder remnant but rather by whether the remnant is closed or left open.

6. The postoperative problems

Laparoscopic cholecystectomies are increasingly common, leading to specific complications like bile duct injuries, retained gallstones, and port site hernias.

Data from the American College of Surgeons National Surgical Quality Improvement Program (ACS-NSQIP) show that open cholecystectomy has higher morbidity, severe morbidity, and mortality rates. Nationwide studies have identified risk factors for complications after laparoscopic cholecystectomy, including advanced age, male gender, comorbidities, and body weight, while surgeon experience and hospital volume were not. Minor biliary and non-biliary complications are often treated conservatively, but major life-threatening complications, like vasculobiliary issues, need prompt attention and management [39, 40].

6.1 Immediately!: Early complications

6.1.1 Vasculobiliary injury

Biliary tree trauma poses a challenge for surgeons due to variable anatomy, limited space, and complication morbidity [41]. Numerous studies on bile duct injuries (BDIs) and cholecystectomies conducted in the past 30 years have shown that bile leak incidence is greater following laparoscopic cholecystectomy (LC) than after open cholecystectomy (OC), with rates of 0.4–0.6% for laparoscopic procedures and 0.1–0.2% for open surgeries [39, 41–43]. Over time, BDIs after LC have decreased to about 0.2% due to increased procedure experience. However, while these injuries are rarer, they are often more severe, particularly biliary and hepatic artery or portal vein injuries following conversion from laparoscopic to open surgery cholecystectomy [42–44].

BDIs pose surgical challenges and significant postoperative complications, including morbidity, up to 35% mortality, and long-term quality of life issues. Therefore, efforts must minimize risks in elective and emergency cases of cholecystectomies [39, 41, 42]. Biliary system injuries during LC often arise from misidentifying the common bile duct (CBD) as the cystic duct, necessitating quick identification and management. Common bile leak sites post-LC are the cystic duct stump and aberrant branches of the hepatic ducts [39, 41]. In recent years, injuries have shifted to more proximal ones in the biliary tract, often causing substance loss and ischemia. These typically result from vascular injuries or energy-driven bile duct lesions. Achieving a critical view of safety (CVS) in LC is crucial for minimizing bile duct injury (BDI) risks from visual perception errors. Studies show recognizing CVS significantly reduces iatrogenic intraoperative complications, thus recommending its routine implementation to prevent BDIs [42, 44, 45].

Effective management of BDIs depends on the severity of the injury to the biliary tract, associated vascular damage, detection time, and underlying mechanisms. A thorough description and diagnosis that covers these aspects is crucial. Various classifications of BDI have emerged over the years, outlining injury subtypes based on severity, biliary tract anatomy, and injury level. Some also include associated vascular injuries at the hepatic hilum. There is no agreement on a "gold standard" classification for BDIs, but several accepted systems will be discussed below [41, 42, 45].

6.1.1.1 Strasberg classification (1995)

In 1995, Strasberg updated the Bismuth classification of BDI to differentiate small bile leaks from the cystic duct of the right sectoral branch and more serious injuries during LC. It categorizes injuries into types A to E, with type E similar to the original Bismuth classification (**Figure 15**) [37, 45]. Type A injuries feature a leak from the cystic duct or small ducts on the liver bed. Type B indicates an occlusion of the aberrant right posterior

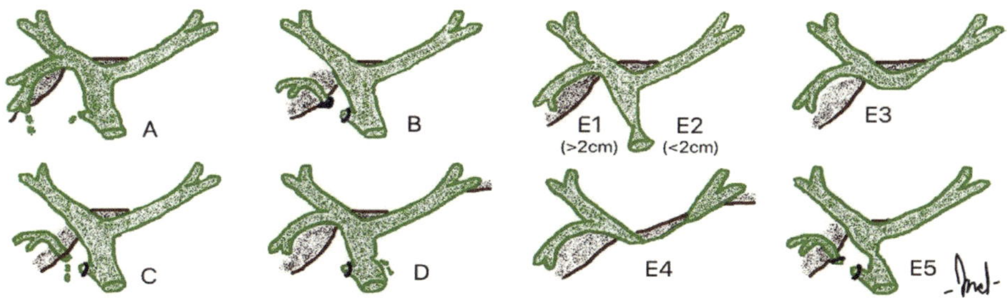

Figure 15.
Strasberg classification [37, 45]. The picture was recreated following the figure published by Chun [45].

hepatic duct, while Type C describes a transection of the right hepatic duct with leakage. These injuries often co-occur with a cystic duct draining into an aberrant hepatic duct. Type D involves an injury to the lateral bile duct affecting less than 50% of its circumference. In contrast, type E injuries are strictures of the hepatic ducts, following the Bismuth classification. A major limitation of the Strasberg classification is its oversight of involvement in vascular issues [37, 41, 45]. The Strasberg classification remains the most widely and universally used classification of BDI to date.

6.1.1.2 Hannover classification (2007)

In 2007, Bektas et al. proposed the Hannover classification after analyzing BDI cases. It categorizes BDIs into five types: A for peripheral bile leaks, B for strictures, C for tangential lateral CHD or CBD injury (further split into four types with vascular injury), D for total CHD transection (also divided into four types), and E for postoperative bile duct stricture without leaks (**Figure 16**). The Hannover classification demonstrates strong statistical significance in linking injury patterns to selected surgical treatments, outperforming other systems that identify fewer patterns. It also associates specific injuries with liver tissue and resection of the hepatic duct bifurcation [45, 46].

6.1.1.3 ATOM: Anatomic, time of detection, and mechanism (2013)

In 2013, the European Association for Endoscopic Surgery (EAES) introduced the ATOM classification, integrating various BDI classifications like Bismuth, Strasberg, and McMahon into one comprehensive system. It combines biliary tract damage, detection timing, and damage mechanisms to classify all possible injuries. The ATOM system seeks to standardize BDI definitions into a unified language [42, 44]. The EAES ATOM classification for BDI includes acronyms: MBD (main bile duct) with levels 1–6; NMBD (non-main bile duct) with O or D and suffixes c or p (%), LS (cm), VBI (RHA, LHA, CHA, PV, MV, Ei, Ep, or L), and Me or ED. Unknown parameters are marked with "?" (**Table 2**) [44].

6.1.2 Fix the vasculobiliary injury

6.1.2.1 When is how - Time-based management

The management of bile duct injury is classified into four categories based on the timing of detection: *immediate*, which refers to the management of injuries identified during the cholecystectomy; *early*, indicating management for injuries detected within less than

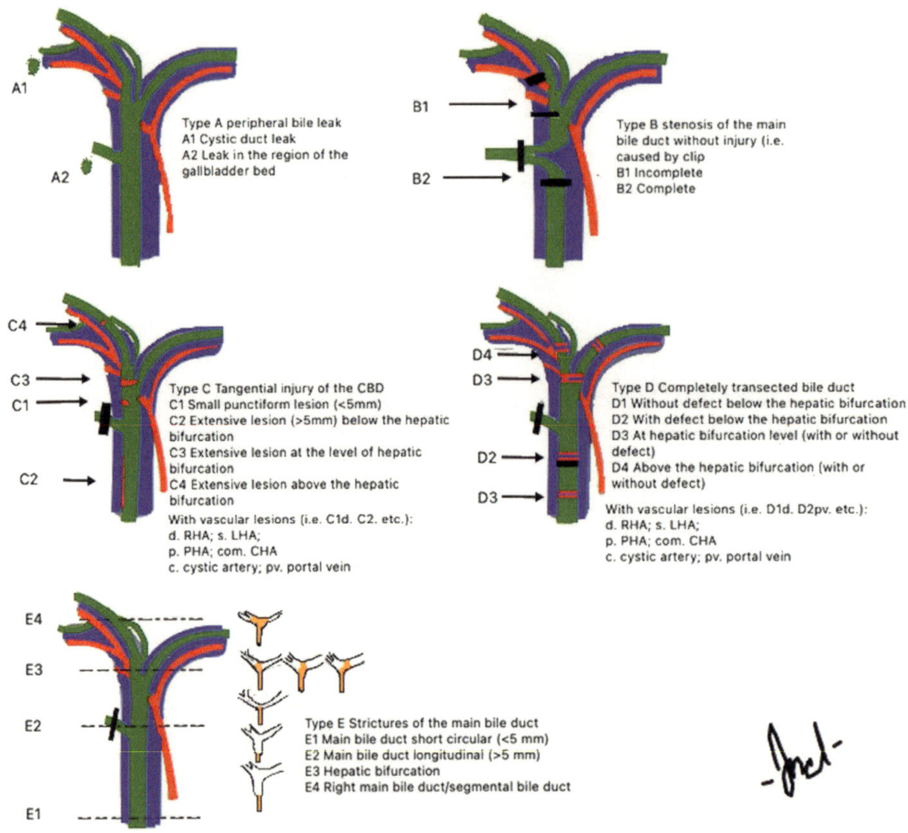

Figure 16.
The Hannover Classification [46].

2 weeks following the procedure; *intermediate*, pertaining to the management of injuries recognized between 2 and 6 weeks post-cholecystectomy; and *late*, denoting management of bile duct injuries detected more than 6 weeks after the surgery [47–49].

Some publications describe early intervention as the management in injuries detected within 72 hours or 7 days after surgery [42, 49].

6.1.2.2 Two sides of the same coins: Major or minor?

The management of bile duct injury is also classified based on the severity: (a) *major injury*, when there is a complete loss of common and/or hepatic bile duct continuity; (b) *minor injury*, which includes injuries caused by electrocautery burns or a partial cut from sharp dissection with shears and are not associated with tissue loss [42].

6.1.2.3 What to do?

6.1.2.3.1 Drain insertion: Drain now, fix later

The insertion of a drain is a safe procedure for managing immediately detected bile duct injury. This intervention may be conducted by a hepatopancreatobiliary (HPB) surgeon or any general surgeon involved in cholecystectomy. The timing of drain utilization can be seen in **Figures 17** and **18**.

Anatomical characteristics							Time of detection			Mechanism	
Anatomic level	Type and extent of injury					Vasculobiliary injury (yes = VBI +) and name of the injured vessel (RHA, LHA, CHA, PV, and MV); (no = VBI -)	Ei (de visu, bile leak, IOC)	Ep	L	Me	ED
	Occlusion		Division								
	C	**P***	**C**	**P***	**LS****						
MBD											
1											
2											
3											
4											
5											
6											
NMBD											

EAES European Association for Endoscopic Surgery.
BDI Bile duct injury.
MBD main biliary duct; NMBD nonmain biliary duct (Luschka duct, aberrant duct, accessory duct).
Level 1, low main BDI ≥ 2 cm distal to the inferior border of superior hepatic confluence.
Level 2, middle main BDI < 2 cm distal to the inferior border of superior hepatic confluence.
Level 3 has a high main BDI involving the superior hepatic confluence, but the left-right communication is preserved.
Level 4, high main BDI involving the superior hepatic confluence, but left-right communication is interrupted.
Level 5, left or right hepatic duct injuries without injury to the superior confluence.
Level 6, isolated segmental hepatic duct injury (right anterior or posterior sectorial).
C, complete; P, partial; LS, loss of substance.
Me, mechanical; ED, energy driven.
VBI, vasculobiliary involvement.
RHA, right hepatic artery; LHA, left hepatic artery; CHA, common hepatic artery; PV, portal vein; MV, marginal vessels.
Ei, early intraoperative; Ep, early postoperative, L late.
*IOC, intraoperative cholangioram.*indicates the percentage of circumference, if known.*
***indicates length, if known [44].*

Table 2.
EAES classification matrix for BDI: For each injury, the surgeon fills out the following matrix: (1) single injury (yes/no); (2) multiple injuries (yes/no). A separate matrix is completed for each injury, as appropriate. For example, an injury caused by an energy-driven (ultrasonic) dissector involving the superior biliary confluence, with interruption of the right and left hepatic ducts, detected intraoperatively during the surgery by the presence of bile, would be classified as MBD 4 C VBI Ei, ED [44].

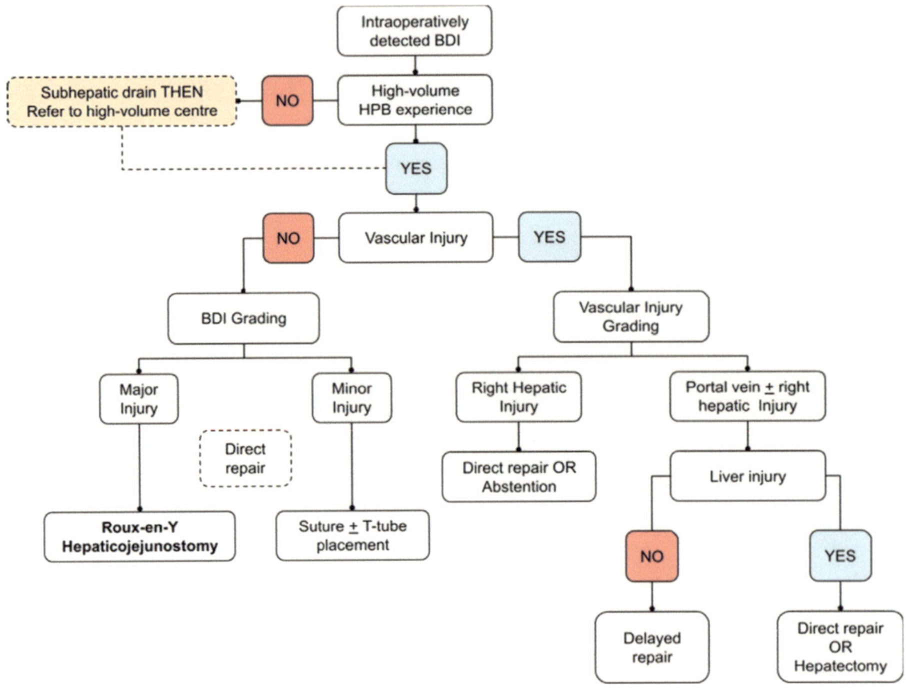

Figure 17.
Management of intraoperatively detected bile duct injury [42].

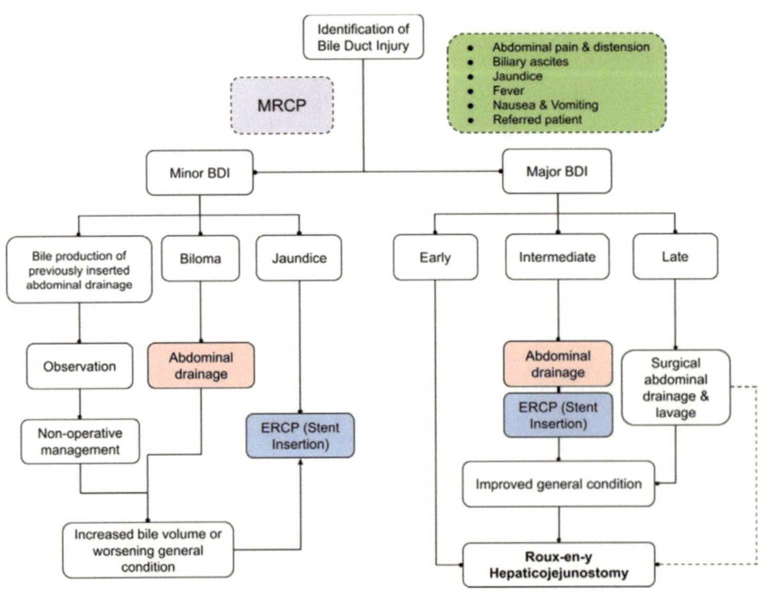

Figure 18.
Management of postoperative bile duct injury [42].

Several types of drain tubes may be utilized for placement into the Morison's pouch or the right subhepatic area, including (1) Penrose drain; (2) nasogastric tube (NGT); (3) Jackson-Pratt drain; and (4) Hemovac drain.

6.1.2.3.2 T-tube

T-tube insertion is commonly performed for minor biliary duct injuries identified intraoperatively. This procedure may occur simultaneously with the placement of an abdominal drain. The primary aim of this intervention is to minimize the risk of strictures at the site of injury in the future [42].

6.1.2.3.3 Endoscopic retrograde cholangio-pancreatography (ERCP)

Endoscopic retrograde cholangiopancreatography (ERCP) is utilized not only as a diagnostic tool but also, in conjunction with stent insertion, as a preferred treatment modality for minor bile duct injuries (BDIs) detected after surgery. This approach allows for the accurate visualization of the bile duct anatomy and the identification of any obstructions or injuries. Inserting a stent can facilitate bile drainage and promote injury healing by maintaining duct patency. Thus, ERCP with stent placement serves as an effective management strategy for addressing minor postoperative bile duct injuries.

6.1.2.3.4 Biliodigestive bypass

The treatment of choice in almost all types of bile duct injury is a biliodigestive bypass, and the most recommended technique of bypass is Roux-en-y hepaticojejunostomy.

For certain types of injury, lowering the hilar plate and performing parenchymal dissection to expose the roof of the confluence and the left intrahepatic duct are necessary.

Monofilament and unbraided sutures are needed, usually 5/0 to 7/0.

6.1.2.4 Summary of BDI classification and management

See **Table 3**.

	Classification			**Management**
	Strasberg	**Hannover**	**ATOM**	
Major	E1 E2 E3 E4 E5	Type C Type D	MBDI 1 MBDI 2 MBDI 3 MBDI 4 MBDI 5 MBDI 6	Roux-en-y Hepaticojejunostomy
Minor	A B C D	Type A Type B Type E	NMBD	ERCP + stent insertion T-tube placement

BDI, bile duct injury.
ATOM, anatomic, time of detection, mechanism.
MBDI, main biliary duct injury.
NMBD, non-main biliary duct.
ERCP, endoscopic retrograde cholangiopancreatography.

Table 3.
Summary of bile duct injury and management.

Risk factors for bleeding in laparoscopic cholecystectomy	
Surgical Factors	• Inadequate training and experience • Rough technique • Improper usage of instruments • Inadequate exposure • Failure to recognize anatomical landmarks • Forceful retraction
Patient-Related	• Acute cholecystitis • Cirrhosis • Portal hypertension • Coagulopathy • Adhesions • Previous surgery • Anatomical abnormalities
Instrument Failures	• Defective instruments

Table 4.
Factors implicated in the causation of bleeding complications [50].

6.1.3 The hemorrhage

Bleeding complications during cholecystectomy are non-biliary issues that can arise and may lead to death if not promptly recognized and managed during the procedure. They constitute up to one-third of major complications in LC and are the leading cause of procedure-related mortality in LC after anaesthesia-related deaths. Studies indicate the bleeding risk in LC is 0.08% compared to 0.54% in open OC. However, uncontrollable intraoperative bleeding from vascular injury occurs in 0.9% to 1.9% of cases [39, 50, 51]. Various factors contribute to bleeding (**Table 4**), with surgeon-related factors being critical, emphasizing proper training. Reports show that surgeons with fewer than 100 cases face more bleeding complications, a trend that diminishes with increased experience [50].

Bleeding during cholecystectomy often comes from the gallbladder bed and is treated with a fibrin-collagen patch and electrocautery. Other bleeding sources, like tangential lesions and cystic artery division, are managed with laparoscopic clips. Rarely, injury to the hepatic artery may necessitate open surgery. Reports also note bleeding from the omentum, and accidental hepatic parenchyma penetration can damage the middle hepatic vein, often near the gallbladder fossa. Studies show that 10 to 15% of cases have a significant branch of the middle hepatic vein adjacent to the gallbladder fossa. In comparison, 6 to 15% have a large vein within 1 mm of the gallbladder bed—preoperative assessment of the middle hepatic vein and gallbladder bed benefits from venous Doppler ultrasonography and CT imaging. Caution is key after dissecting the hepatocystic triangle and confirming the CVS to minimize the risk of bleeding complications in LC [39, 50, 51].

6.2 Too little, too late: Delayed complications

6.2.1 Gallstone spillage

Gallbladder perforation with stones spilling into the peritoneal cavity is a common complication in cholecystectomy, especially in acute cholecystitis. Reports of complications from spilled stones during open cholecystectomy are rare, as spillage is easily managed, and stones can typically be retrieved. However, perforation during laparoscopic cholecystectomy (LC) is more frequent and more challenging to control, with rates of 10–30%. Causes include excessive traction, instrument puncture, and removal of a distended gallbladder through a trocar site. This complicates the detection and retrieval of spilled stones, increasing complications during laparoscopy [39, 40].

Gallstone spillage occurs intraoperatively but can lead to complications weeks to years later, including abscesses, fistulas, liver abscesses, and bacteraemia. Symptomatic stones often reside in the peri-hepatic area, especially Morrison's pouch and operative port sites. Due to rare complications, open procedures during gallbladder perforation are discouraged. Instead, attempt to retrieve stones with suction, forceps, and irrigation. It is essential to document the incident and inform the patient, as spilled stones may resemble hepatic and peritoneal metastases [39, 40, 52].

6.2.2 Did you miss something?: Remnant gallbladder and cystic duct stones remnant

The persistence of post-cholecystectomy symptoms may result from retained stones or new stones in a remnant gallbladder. Up to 30% of post-cholecystectomy pain may involve stone disease in a remnant cystic duct or gallbladder. It can be challenging to identify if a stone persists in a cystic duct remnant or if there's a relapse of lithiasis. Incomplete gallbladder removal after open cholecystectomy is rare, but the laparoscopic era shows slightly higher rates of unintentional incomplete removal. Reports typically focus on surgically managed patients, yet anecdotal evidence suggests incomplete removal is more frequent in laparoscopic procedures, occurring in up to 13.3% of cases, likely due to the prevalence of subtotal cholecystectomy during this period [39, 53].

Some surgeons intentionally leave the gallbladder pouch sutured closed during laparoscopic subtotal cholecystectomy. This differs from open subtotal cholecystectomy, where the gallbladder's posterior wall remains attached to the liver, and the cystic duct is secured with a purse-string technique [39]. Reasons for incomplete resection include poor visualization of the gallbladder fossa, adhesions, inflammation, excessive bleeding, or complex gallbladder morphology like congenital duplication or an hourglass configuration due to adenomyomatosis [53].

Alternative laparoscopic approaches to subtotal cholecystectomy are more convenient, but they increase the risk of relapsing lithiasis. In one study, cystic duct remnant lithiasis occurred in 4.19% of laparoscopic subtotal cholecystectomy cases, compared to 0.02% in conventional laparoscopic cholecystectomy. Both laparoscopic and open techniques have been used for resection of the gallbladder and cystic duct remnants. Advanced endoscopic methods could provide even less invasive management [39, 53].

6.3 Post-cholecystectomy diarrhea

Cholecystectomy causes small changes in enterohepatic circulation. Unlike Crohn's disease, it does not cause actual malabsorption. [54] Ileal bile acids are absorbed to activate ileal Farnesoid X receptor (FXR), which in turn induces the transcription of fibroblast growth factor 19 (FGF19). This can activate hepatic FXR and stop the activity of cytochrome P450 7A1 (CYP7A1), hence decreasing the production of bile acid synthesis. This mechanism is called the negative feedback mechanism in normal conditions [55].

About 2.1–57.2% of post-cholecystectomy patients experience diarrhea, which is caused by the increased entry of bile acid into the colon [56]. It happens because the negative feedback mechanism in bile acid synthesis is disrupted, leading to a hepatic overproduction of bile acids. Bile acids can induce fluid secretion and increase mucosal permeability of the colon, causing an increase of peristalsis.

7. Adaptation and dysfunction without gallbladder

Some patients after cholecystectomy might experience post-cholecystectomy syndrome, which is a dysfunction of the sphincter of Oddi caused by non-calculous obstructive disorder, which decreases bile passage and pancreatic juice outflow into the duodenum. Symptoms could vary, such as stomach upset, nausea, vomiting, gaseous distention, diarrhea, or pain at the right abdomen, especially after eating a fatty meal. The pain may be recurrent, of moderate to severe intensity, and lasts for more than 20 minutes [57, 58].

The absence of the gallbladder causes the passage of hepatic bile to increase into the duodenum and the gallbladder-independent enterohepatic circulation of biliary cholesterol, bilirubin, and bile acid. This results in an increased concentration of bile acids in the hepatocytes, decreases the accumulation and excretory function of the liver, and helps in increased absorption of biliary cholesterol in the small intestine. Due to all these alterations in enterohepatic circulation, lithogenic hepatic bile is formed, which causes stones to form in the bile ducts. An increase in the gallbladder's independent output of biliary cholesterol and the concentration of total bile acids in duodenal bile causes the precipitation of cholesterol monohydrate crystals in the duodenal lumen [57].

Acknowledgements

ChatGPT was used for its assistance in correcting grammar and rephrasing English sentences.

The authors thank Azzahra Fadhilah, MD, for her invaluable assistance in organizing the manuscript. Her attention to detail enhances the presentation of this chapter.

Conflict of interest

The authors declare no conflict of interest.

DOI: http://dx.doi.org/10.5772/intechopen.1010679

Author details

Vania Myralda Giamour Marbun[1*], Indah Jamtani[2], Karl Heinz Leonhardt Rowika[3] and Nafilla Nesantya Sabatini[3]

1 Department of Surgery, Universitas Indonesia – Cipto Mangunkusumo Hospital, Jakarta, Indonesia

2 Department of Surgery, Universitas Indonesia – Fatmawati Hospital, Jakarta, Indonesia

3 Department of Surgery, Universitas Indonesia, Jakarta, Indonesia

*Address all correspondence to: vania.myralda@gmail.com

References

[1] Imber G. Genius on the Edge: The Bizarre Double Life of Dr. William Stewart Halsted. 1st ed. New York: USA: Kaplan Publishing; 2010

[2] Sparkman RS. 100th anniversary of the first cholecystectomy. Archives of Surgery (Chicago, Ill. : 1960). 1982;**117**:1525. DOI: 10.1001/archsurg.1982.01380360001001

[3] Traverso LW. Carl Langenbuch and the first cholecystectomy. American Journal of Surgery. 1976;**132**:81-82. DOI: 10.1016/0002-9610(76)90295-6

[4] De U. Evolution of cholecystectomy: A tribute to Carl August Langenbuch. The Indian Journal of Surgery. 2004;**66**(2):66. ISSN 0972-2068

[5] Metzger A. History of laparoscopic cholecystectomy. In: Büchler MW, Frei E, Klaiber C, Krähenbühl L, editors. Prog. Surg. Vol. 22. S. Bern: Karger AG; 1996. pp. 25-31. DOI: 10.1159/000425265

[6] Hundt M, Wu CY, Young M. Anatomy, Abdomen and Pelvis: Biliary Ducts. StatPearls, Treasure Island (FL): StatPearls Publishing; 2025

[7] Desmet V, Roskams T, De Vos R. Normal anatomy. In: Gastroenterol. Hepatol. Gallbladder Bile Ducts. 6th ed. United States: Current Medicine; 1995

[8] Hundt M, Basit H, John S. Physiology, bile secretion. In: StatPearls. Treasure Island (FL): StatPearls Publishing; 2025

[9] Esteller A. Physiology of bile secretion. World Journal of Gastroenterology. 2008;**14**:5641-5649. DOI: 10.3748/wjg.14.5641

[10] Nagashree MV, Chandragirish S, Raghavendra DR, Chandrakala SP, Pare VS. Study of normal anatomy and variations in gall bladder. International Journal of Health Sciences. 2022;**6**:11479-11491. DOI: 10.53730/ijhs.v6nS6.13179

[11] Harlaftis N, Gray SW, Skandalakis JE. Multiple gallbladders. Surgery, Gynecology & Obstetrics. 1977;**145**:928-934

[12] Gündüz N, Doğan MB, Alacagöz M, Yağbasan M, Orhan Söylemez UP, Atalay B. Anatomical variations of cystic duct insertion and their relationship with choledocholithiasis: An MRCP study. Egyptian Journal of Radiology and Nuclear Medicine. 2021;**52**:202. DOI: 10.1186/s43055-021-00579-x

[13] Turner MA, Fulcher AS. The cystic duct: Normal anatomy and disease processes. Radiographics. 2001;**21**:3-22. DOI: 10.1148/radiographics.21.1.g01ja093

[14] Andall RG, Matusz P, du Plessis M, Ward R, Tubbs RS, Loukas M. The clinical anatomy of cystic artery variations: A review of over 9800 cases. Surgical and Radiologic Anatomy : SRA. 2016;**38**:529-539. DOI: 10.1007/s00276-015-1600-y

[15] Triantafyllou G, Belimezakis N, Lyros O, Tsakotos G, Botis G, Piagkou M. Surgical anatomy of the cystic artery: A systematic review with meta-analysis. Annals of Anatomy = Anatomischer Anzeiger. 2025;**257**:152343. DOI: 10.1016/j.aanat.2024.152343

[16] Jones MW, Guay E, Deppen JG. Open cholecystectomy. In: StatPearls. Treasure Island (FL): StatPearls Publishing; 2025

[17] Ellison EC, Zollinger RM, Pawlik TM, Vaccaro PS, Bitans M, Baker AS, et al. Chapter 70 cholecystectomy, open

retrograde technique. In: Zollingers Atlas Surg. Oper. 11th ed. New York: McGraw-Hill Education; 2022. pp. 262-267

[18] Skandalakis LJ, Skandalakis JE, Panajiotis NS. Chapter 14: Extrahepatic biliary tract. In: Surg. Anat. Tech. Pocket Man. Cham: Springer International Publishing; 2021. pp. 593-642. DOI: 10.1007/978-3-030-51313-9

[19] Cameron J, Sandonne C. Atlas of Gastrointestinal Surgery. 2nd ed. Shelton: People's Medical Publishing House; 2014

[20] Alkatout I, Mettler L, Maass N, Noé G-K, Elessawy M. Abdominal anatomy in the context of port placement and trocars. Journal of the Turkish German Gynecological Association. 2015;**16**:241-251. DOI: 10.5152/jtgga.2015.0148

[21] Marc Rafols, Navid Ajabshir, and Kfir Ben-David. Fundamentals of General Surgery. Cham: Springer International Publishing; 2018. DOI: 10.1007/978-3-319-75656-1

[22] Dahmane R, Morjane A, Starc A. Anatomy and surgical relevance of Rouviere's sulcus. The Scientific World Journal. 2013;**2013**:254287. DOI: 10.1155/2013/254287

[23] Ragavan S, Muraleedharan A, Bage NN, et al. Rouviere's sulcus: an overemphasized accessory sulcus or an underemphasized normal sulcus? Surgical and Radiologic Anatomy. Heidelberg, Germany: Springer; 2020;**42**(9):1447-1448. DOI: 10.1007/s00276-020-02555-y

[24] Abdelfattah MR. The laparoscopic anatomy of Rouviere's sulcus. Open Access Surgery. 2021;**14**:67-71. DOI: 10.2147/OAS.S341710

[25] Voruganti MR, Mohammed N, Gurrala RC, Chowdary GH, Devarakonda L. Rouviere's Sulcus: Anatomy and its Clinical Significance in Laparoscopic Cholecystectomy. World Journal of Laparoscopic Surgery. 2023;**16**(1):4-7

[26] Sebastian M, Sebastian A, Rudnicki J. The evaluation of B-SAFE and ultrasonographic landmarks in safe orientation during laparoscopic cholecystectomy. Wideochir Inne Tech Maloinwazyjne. Warsaw, Poland: Polish Medical Society; Dec 2020;**15**(4):546-552. DOI: 10.5114/wiitm.2020.100972

[27] Schendel J, Ball C, Dixon E, Sutherland F. Prevalence of anatomic landmarks for orientation during elective laparoscopic cholecystectomies. Surgical Endoscopy. 2020;**34**:3508-3512. DOI: 10.1007/s00464-019-07131-z

[28] Gupta V, Jain G. The R4U planes for the zonal demarcation for safe laparoscopic cholecystectomy. World Journal of Surgery. 2021;**45**:1096-1101. DOI: 10.1007/s00268-020-05908-1

[29] Mischinger H-J, Wagner D, Kornprat P, Bacher H, Werkgartner G. The "Critical View of Safety (CVS)" cannot be applied—What to do? Strategies to avoid bile duct injuries. European Surgery. 2021;**53**:99-105. DOI: 10.1007/s10353-020-00660-1

[30] Obonna GC, Obonna MC. Role of indocyanine green in laparoscopic cholecystectomy. World Journal of Laparoscopic Surgery. 2020;**13**:1-3. DOI: 10.5005/jp-journals-10033-1388

[31] Nouh MA, Salah Helmy A, Abbas M, Nasr M, Emad Esmat M, Adel Aziz S, et al. Indocyanine green as an alternative to intraoperative cholangiogram to delineate extrahepatic biliary tract in laparoscopic cholecystectomy. Surgery, Gastroenterology and Oncology. 2024;**29**:219. DOI: 10.21614/sgo-698

[32] Cárdenas G, Fornaguera I, Díaz Del Gobbo R, Ginestà C. Direct gallbladder indocyanine green injection technique to achieve critical view of safety in laparoscopic cholecystectomy. Cirugía Española (English Edition). 2021;**99**:678-682. DOI: 10.1016/j.cireng.2021.09.001

[33] Nagata S, Kai S, Korenaga D, Mori M, Toyota S, Orita H. Analysis of bailout procedure in laparoscopic cholecystectomy for acute cholecystitis. Durham, NC, USA: Research Square; 2021. DOI: 10.21203/rs.3.rs-257094/v1

[34] Abe T, Oshita A, Fujikuni N, Hattori M, Kobayashi T, Hanada K, et al. Efficacy of bailout surgery for preventing intraoperative biliary injury in acute cholecystitis. Surgical Endoscopy. 2023;**37**:2595-2603. DOI: 10.1007/s00464-022-09755-0

[35] Iwashita Y, Hibi T, Ohyama T, Umezawa A, Takada T, Strasberg SM, et al. Delphi consensus on bile duct injuries during laparoscopic cholecystectomy: An evolutionary cul-de-sac or the birth pangs of a new technical framework? Journal of Hepato-biliary-pancreatic Sciences. 2017;**24**:591-602. DOI: 10.1002/jhbp.503

[36] Henneman D, Da Costa DW, Vrouenraets BC, Van Wagensveld BA, Lagarde SM. Laparoscopic partial cholecystectomy for the difficult gallbladder: A systematic review. Surgical Endoscopy. 2013;**27**:351-358. DOI: 10.1007/s00464-012-2458-2

[37] Strasberg SM, Hertl M, Soper NJ. An analysis of the problem of biliary injury during laparoscopic cholecystectomy. Journal of the American College of Surgeons. 1995;**180**:101-125

[38] Strasberg SM, Pucci MJ, Brunt ML, Deziel DJ. Subtotal cholecystectomy–"Fenestrating" vs "Reconstituting" subtypes and the prevention of bile duct injury: Definition of the optimal procedure in difficult operative conditions. Journal of the American College of Surgeons. 2016;**222**:89-96. DOI: 10.1016/j.jamcollsurg.2015.09.019

[39] Lee MK IV, Vollmer CM Jr. Postcholecystectomy problems. In: Blumgarts Surg. Liver Biliary Tract Pancreas. 6th ed. Vol. 1. Philadelphia: Elsevier, Inc.; 2017. p. 13

[40] Radunovic M, Lazovic R, Popovic N, Magdelinic M, Bulajic M, Radunovic L, et al. Complications of laparoscopic cholecystectomy: Our experience from a retrospective analysis. Open Access Macedonian Journal of Medical Sciences. 2016;**4**:641-646. DOI: 10.3889/oamjms.2016.128

[41] Moghul F, Kashyap S. Bile duct injury. In: StatPearls. Treasure Island (FL): StatPearls Publishing; 2025

[42] de'Angelis N, Catena F, Memeo R, Coccolini F, Martínez-Pérez A, Romeo OM, et al. WSES guidelines for the detection and management of bile duct injury during cholecystectomy. World Journal of Emergency Surgery : WJES. 2020;**2021**(16):30. DOI: 10.1186/s13017-021-00369-w

[43] Zidan MHE-D, Seif-Eldeen M, Ghazal AA, Refaie M. Post-cholecystectomy bile duct injuries: A retrospective cohort study. BMC Surgery. 2024;**24**:8. DOI: 10.1186/s12893-023-02301-2

[44] Fingerhut A, Dziri C, Garden OJ, Gouma D, Millat B, Neugebauer E, et al. ATOM, the all-inclusive, nominal EAES classification of bile duct injuries during cholecystectomy. Surgical Endoscopy.

2013;**27**:4608-4619. DOI: 10.1007/s00464-013-3081-6

[45] Chun K. Recent classifications of the common bile duct injury. Korean Journal of Hepato-biliary-pancreatic Surgery. 2014;**18**:69-72. DOI: 10.14701/kjhbps.2014.18.3.69

[46] Bektas H, Schrem H, Winny M, Klempnauer J. Surgical treatment and outcome of iatrogenic bile duct lesions after cholecystectomy and the impact of different clinical classification systems. The British Journal of Surgery. 2007;**94**:1119-1127. DOI: 10.1002/bjs.5752

[47] Lalisang TJM, Situmorang I, Ibrahim F, Widianto P, Marbun VMG. Management of post-cholecystectomy bile duct injuries without operative mortality at Jakarta tertiary hospital in Indonesia – A cross-sectional study. Annals of Medicine and Surgery. 2021;**62**:211-215. DOI: 10.1016/j.amsu.2021.01.012

[48] Manivasagam SS, Chandra JN, Khera D, Aradhya PS, Hiremath AM. Optimal timing of surgical repair after bile duct injury: A systematic review and meta-analysis. Cureus. 2024. DOI: 10.7759/cureus.53507

[49] Rystedt JML, Kleeff J, Salvia R, Besselink MG, Prasad R, Lesurtel M, et al. Post cholecystectomy bile duct injury: Early, intermediate or late repair with hepaticojejunostomy – An E-AHPBA multi-center study. HPB. 2019;**21**:1641-1647. DOI: 10.1016/j.hpb.2019.04.003

[50] Kaushik R. Bleeding complications in laparoscopic cholecystectomy: Incidence, mechanisms, prevention and management. Journal of Minimal Access Surgery. 2010;**6**:59-65. DOI: 10.4103/0972-9941.68579

[51] Rajeeth G, Tilakaratne S, Siriwardana RC. The hidden threat of uncontrollable bleeding from the gallbladder bed during laparoscopic cholecystectomy. International Journal of Surgery Case Reports. 2023;**112**:108957. DOI: 10.1016/j.ijscr.2023.108957

[52] Perrotti G, O'Moore P, Kirton O. Hey, you forgot something! The Management of Symptomatic Retained Gallstones. Surgery in Practice and Science. 2022;**8**:100052. DOI: 10.1016/j.sipas.2021.100052

[53] Chowbey P, Sharma A, Goswami A, Afaque Y, Najma K, Baijal M, et al. Residual gallbladder stones after cholecystectomy: A literature review. Journal of Minimal Access Surgery. 2015;**11**:223-230. DOI: 10.4103/0972-9941.158156

[54] Huang R-L, Huang W-K, Xiao X-Y, Ma L-F, Gu H-Z-R, Yang G-P. Diagnosis and treatment of post-cholecystectomy diarrhoea. World Journal of Gastrointestinal Surgery. 2023;**15**:2398-2405. DOI: 10.4240/wjgs.v15.i11.2398

[55] Farrugia A, Arasaradnam R. Bile acid diarrhoea: Pathophysiology, diagnosis and management. Frontline Gastroenterology. 2021;**12**:500-507. DOI: 10.1136/flgastro-2020-101436

[56] Farrugia A, Attard JA, Hanmer S, Bullock S, McKay S, Al-Azzawi M, et al. Rates of bile acid diarrhoea after cholecystectomy: A multicentre audit. World Journal of Surgery. 2021;**45**:2447-2453. DOI: 10.1007/s00268-021-06147-8

[57] Jaiswal P, Jaiswal BK. Physiological changes after cholecystectomy. Indian Journal of Applied Research. 2016;**6**

[58] Zackria R, Lopez RA. Postcholecystectomy syndrome. In: StatPearls. Treasure Island (FL): StatPearls Publishing; 2025

Chapter 5

Mirizzi Syndrome and Its Management

Karamveer Singh, Arunkumar V, Amit Gupta, Satish Ammapalem and Monisha Selvarasu

Abstract

Mirizzi syndrome is an uncommon complication of chronic gallstone disease, characterized by the impaction of a gallstone into the gallbladder neck or cystic duct, leading to bile duct obstruction and potential fistula formation. This condition, first described by Pablo Luis Mirizzi, results from external compression of the bile duct due to gallstone impaction, often accompanied by inflammation, fibrosis, and tissue necrosis. The syndrome is divided into various types on the basis of the presence and severity of cholecystobiliary or cholecystoenteric fistulas, with type I involving external compression and types II–V involving fistula formation. Clinically, Mirizzi syndrome presents with symptoms such as right upper quadrant pain, fever, and jaundice, though the classic triad is seen in only 44–71% of cases. The diagnosis relies on imaging modalities, including ultrasonography, CT, magnetic resonance cholangiopancreatography (MRCP), and endoscopic retrograde cholangiopancreatography (ERCP), with ERCP being the gold standard despite its invasiveness. Surgical management remains the primary treatment, with open cholecystectomy traditionally preferred. However, laparoscopic and robot-assisted techniques combined with endoscopic techniques are increasingly utilized, particularly for complex cases, offering minimally invasive options with improved outcomes. Endoscopic interventions, such as ERCP, play a complementary role, especially in preoperative biliary decompression or stone extraction. Despite advancements in diagnostic and therapeutic techniques, Mirizzi syndrome is often diagnosed intraoperatively, underscoring the need for surgical expertise and a multidisciplinary approach. Tailored management strategies, including subtotal cholecystectomy or hepaticojejunostomy, are essential to address anatomical distortions and minimize complications. This review highlights the evolving understanding and management of Mirizzi syndrome, emphasizing the importance of individualized treatment plans to ensure optimal patient outcomes.

Keywords: Mirizzi syndrome, gallstone, cholecystobiliary fistula, cholecystoenteric fistula, hepaticojejunostomy

1. Introduction

Mirizzi syndrome (MS) is an uncommon condition that arises as a complication of prolonged gallstone disease. It develops when a gallstone becomes lodged in the neck or infundibulum (Hartmann's pouch) of the gallbladder or within the cystic duct, causing external compression and obstruction of the common bile duct (CBD) or common hepatic duct (CHD) [1]. Over time, the persistent presence of gallstones and associated chronic inflammation can result in tissue necrosis, fibrosis, and the eventual formation of a cholecysto-choledochal fistula [2].

This condition is named after Pablo Luis Mirizzi, an Argentine surgeon, although he was not the first to document the syndrome. Earlier descriptions were provided in 1905 by Kehr and in 1908 by Ruge, who identified it as a partial blockage resulting from a chronically lodged gallstone and accompanying inflammation [3]. Mirizzi coined the term "hepatic duct syndrome" in 1948 in relation to cholelithiasis and cholecystitis. He suggested that the mechanical blockage of the gallbladder, along with inflammation of the infundibulum, led to the constriction of what was thought to be a "muscular sphincter" in the common hepatic duct. However, modern understanding has clarified that no such sphincter exists, and the condition is instead caused by external compression of the CHD or CBD due to an impacted stone [4].

2. Pathophysiology

Mirizzi syndrome arises due to external compression of the bile duct caused by a gallstone lodged in Hartmann's pouch or the gallbladder infundibulum and the cystic duct. The impaction of the stone triggers acute or chronic inflammation, which can progress to cholecystobiliary or cholecystoenteric fistula. A predisposing factor for this condition is a lengthy cystic duct, which is parallel to the bile duct and inserts at a low position into the bile duct [5–7]. Prolonged gallstone impaction often results in recurrent attacks of acute cholecystitis. In an early stage, the gallbladder may become enlarged with thickened, inflamed walls. Over time, it tends to shrink and become atrophic, with walls that may thicken and become fibrotic. In advanced stages, the gallbladder walls may either thin out or remain thickened, sometimes adhering tightly to the stones within [8].

When the inflamed gallbladder lies near the bile duct and adheres to it over a period of time, the resulting inflammation and fibrosis can cause bile duct obstruction. Prolonged pressure from the gallstone can lead to tissue necrosis, causing damage and eventually eroding into the common hepatic duct, forming a cholecystobiliary fistula. This is often supported by the presence of a gallstone lodged at the fistulous site [9]. Although rare, retained cystic duct stones following cholecystectomy can also contribute to Mirizzi syndrome. Additionally, with the increased use of bailout techniques, stones in the remnant or neo-gallbladder can lead to the development of this condition.

3. Classification

The initial classification of Mirizzi syndrome was proposed by Corlette et al. in 1975, which divided the condition into two types on the basis of the presence and severity of cholecystobiliary fistulas. However, the most widely followed classification, still in use today, was introduced by McSherry et al. in 1982 on the basis of findings from ERCP. Mirizzi syndrome is classified into two primary types: Type I involves a gallstone becoming trapped in the gallbladder neck, causing external compression of the bile duct, while type II occurs when the erosion of the stone results in the development of a cholecystobiliary fistula [10].

In 1989, Csendes et al. proposed a more detailed classification system for Mirizzi syndrome, particularly focusing on cases involving cholecystobiliary fistulas. This classification is on the basis of the presence and severity of the fistula and is divided into four types [11]:

Mirizzi type I (11% of cases): A gallstone trapped in the neck, infundibulum, or cystic duct of the gallbladder causes compression externally to the common hepatic duct without fistula formation.

Mirizzi type II (41% of cases): A fistula involving less than one-third of the circumference of the common bile duct.

Mirizzi type III (44% of cases): The fistula involves between one-third and two-thirds of the common bile duct's circumference.

Mirizzi type IV (4% of cases): The common bile duct wall is completely destroyed due to the fistula.

This classification provides a more comprehensive understanding of the condition, particularly in cases where fistulas are present (**Figure 1**).

In 2007, Csendes introduced type V to the classification of Mirizzi syndrome, a category later confirmed by Beltran and Csendes in 2008 [7]. This addition was based on a case who had Mirizzi syndrome and features of intestinal obstruction due to gallstone ileus, demonstrating that the condition could progress beyond cholecystobiliary fistulas to involve more complex complications. Persistent inflammation around Calot's triangle can lead to the development of fistulas not only involving the bile ducts but also neighboring organs through similar pathological processes [7]. Type V is characterized by the presence of a cholecystoenteric fistula and is divided into:

Type Va: Cholecystoenteric fistula without gallstone ileus.

Type Vb: Cholecystoenteric fistula with gallstone ileus.

In 2012, Beltran proposed a streamlined classification system with three primary categories [5]:

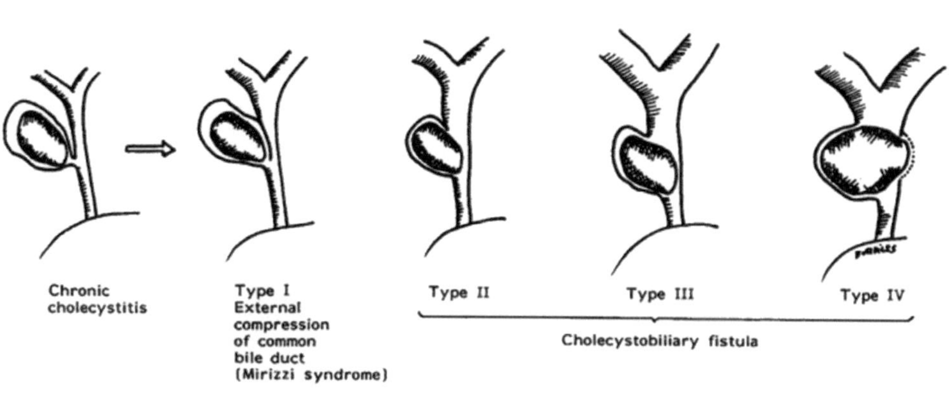

Figure 1.
Csendes classification [11].

Mirizzi type I: Compression of the bile duct due to external pressure as a result of chronic or acute inflammation and a gallstone lodged in Hartmann's pouch or the infundibulum, aligning with type I in both McSherry's and Csendes' classifications.

Mirizzi type IIa: A cholecystobiliary fistula affecting less than half of the bile duct's diameter.

Mirizzi type IIb: A cholecystobiliary fistula affecting more than half of the bile duct's diameter.

Mirizzi type IIIa: A combination of a cholecystobiliary fistula and a cholecystoenteric fistula without features of gallstone ileus.

Mirizzi type IIIb: A cholecystobiliary fistula accompanied by a cholecystoenteric fistula with features of gallstone ileus.

Payá-Llorente et al. refined Beltran's 2012 classification in 2017, suggesting that a cholecystoenteric fistula should be considered a subtype rather than a separate type

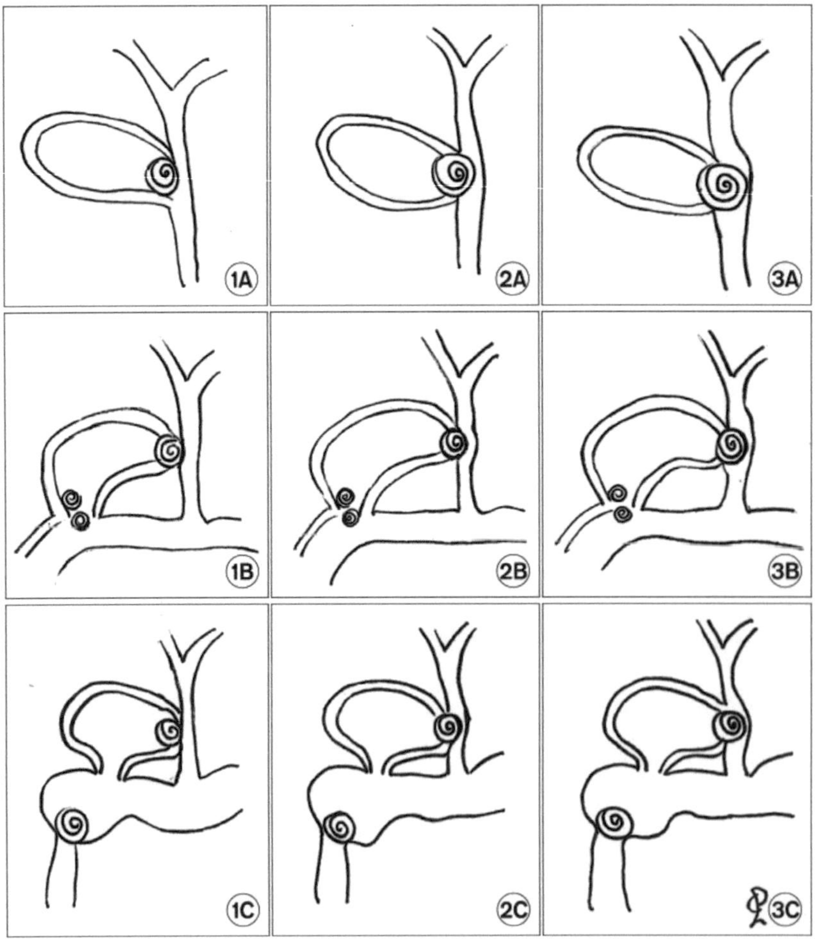

Figure 2.
Payá-Llorente et al.'s revised classification [12].

of Mirizzi syndrome. Their system includes three main types, each with subcategories A, B, and C:

Type 1: The common hepatic duct (CHD) is compressed externally, typically due to a gallstone or an inflammatory process.

Type 2: A fistula forms between the gallbladder and bile duct, affecting less than half of the common bile duct's (CBD) circumference.

Type 3: A fistula develops between the gallbladder and bile duct, involving more than half of the common bile duct's (CBD) circumference.

Subtypes:

A: Absence of a cholecystoenteric fistula.

B: Presence of a cholecystoenteric fistula without features of gallstone ileus.

C: Presence of a cholecystoenteric fistula with features of gallstone ileus (**Figure 2**) [12].

4. Clinical features

Mirizzi syndrome is more frequently observed in women, with symptoms typically appearing between the ages of 21 and 90. Common clinical features include upper abdominal pain on the right side, fever, and jaundice, although only 44–71% of patients exhibit all three symptoms simultaneously. Pain is the most frequently observed symptom, occurring in 54–100% of cases, while jaundice is reported in 24–100% of instances, and cholangitis affects 6–35% of patients. Approximately 33% of patients may present with acute cholecystitis [12–14], and in rare instances, acute pancreatitis may also occur [15].

Patients diagnosed with Mirizzi syndrome are at a heightened risk (5–28%) of gallbladder malignancy, likely due to long-standing biliary stasis causing continuous inflammation in the region. While CA 19-9 levels can assist in differentiating Mirizzi syndrome from gallbladder cancer, they are not entirely reliable, as increased CA 19-9 levels have also been observed in cases of Mirizzi syndrome without malignant changes [16].

If a gallstone migrates from the gallbladder through a cholecystoenteric fistula and becomes lodged in the gastrointestinal tract, it leads to mechanical bowel obstruction, called gallstone ileus. This condition typically presents with symptoms such as abdominal pain, vomiting, and not being able to pass flatus or feces [17]. Rigler's triad is a classic diagnostic indicator for gallstone ileus, which includes the presence of pneumobilia, features of small bowel obstruction, and the ectopic gallstone, typically located in the right iliac fossa [18]. Sometimes a stone may get impacted in the duodenum or pylorus, leading to symptoms of gastric outlet obstruction called Bouveret syndrome, a variant of gallstone ileus [19].

5. Laboratory investigations

Complete blood counts and liver function tests are routinely done in all patients presenting with the above symptoms, and they may show leukocytosis, hyperbilirubinemia, elevated transaminases, and alkaline phosphatase levels. Increased white blood cell (WBC) counts are usually associated with concurrent acute cholecystitis, cholangitis, or pancreatitis [6]. Carbohydrate antigen 19-9 (CA 19-9) levels can be raised, particularly in patients with Mirizzi syndrome type II or more advanced stages. CA 19-9 is a type of glycoprotein associated with various cancers, such as those of the pancreas, biliary tract, or stomach. It is also naturally produced by normal pancreatic tissue, bile duct epithelial cells, and salivary mucosa. Therefore, raised serum CA 19-9 levels should be interpreted carefully in cases of biliary obstruction to avoid misdiagnosing benign conditions as biliary tract or gallbladder cancer. In our view, routine measurement of CA 19-9 in patients with biliary sepsis lacks clinical utility [20].

6. Diagnosis

The diagnosis of Mirizzi syndrome on clinical grounds and laboratory findings is difficult. Preoperatively recognizing Mirizzi syndrome will avoid serious pitfalls intraoperatively, such as

1. Dense adhesions in the hepatoduodenal ligament can cause injury to the common bile duct.

2. The unrecognized Mirizzi syndrome can lead to biliary leak postoperatively.

3. Gross appearance can mimic malignancy, which may lead to unnecessary radical surgery for a benign cause.

Hence, radiological diagnosis is prudent to avoid these complications. The typical diagnostic signs would be dilatation of the common hepatic duct above the level of gallstone impaction in the cystic duct and normal width of the common bile duct below the stone impaction. Since the syndrome does not always show all these typical features, the radiological diagnosis is sometimes undetectable.

Diagnostic tools for identifying Mirizzi syndrome include abdominal ultrasonography, contrast-enhanced computed tomography (CECT), magnetic resonance cholangiopancreatography (MRCP), and endoscopic retrograde cholangiopancreatography (ERCP).

6.1 Abdominal ultrasonography

Ultrasonography is regarded as a first-line diagnostic tool for evaluating biliary pathologies. It can detect conditions such as gallstones, cholecystitis, and signs suggestive of Mirizzi syndrome, including an atrophy of the gallbladder, the presence of one big or numerous small impacted gallstones at the infundibulum or cystic duct with dilatation of the common hepatic duct and a normal distal common bile duct, or a thickened gallbladder wall due to acute cholecystitis.

The difficulty of diagnosing Mirizzi syndrome by sonography is because of the close proximity of the cystic and common bile ducts [21]. However, the sensitivity of ultrasound for diagnosing Mirizzi syndrome varies, reaching up to 77.8%, while its specificity is relatively low at 29% [22].

6.2 Computed tomography

The sensitivity of CT scans in detecting Mirizzi syndrome ranges from 31 to 50%, while its specificity is notably higher at 97%. However, CT imaging often fails to clearly identify biliary calculi. Only 79% of gallstones detected by sonography are recognized on CT [23]. Despite this limitation, CT is valuable for ruling out extraluminal causes of biliary compression, such as biliary or hepatic neoplasm in the porta hepatis or any other sources of biliary obstruction. However, there is no clear evidence that CT provides additional significant information than ultrasonography [21]. Additionally, the presence of pneumobilia in a CT scan, in the absence of prior biliary procedures, may indicate the existence of a cholecystobiliary or cholecystoenteric fistula (**Figure 3**) [24].

6.3 Magnetic resonance cholangiopancreatography

MRCP works on the principle that stationary fluids are hyperintense on heavily T2-weighted images. It is the most favored noninvasive imaging technique for assessing biliary anatomy and diagnosing Mirizzi syndrome. However, MRCP findings for Mirizzi syndrome can sometimes be mistaken for gallbladder malignancy, cholangiocarcinoma, metastatic disease in the hilum, or acute cholecystitis. In such instances, combining MRCP with CT imaging can help reduce these false-positive results [24].

Key MRCP findings for Mirizzi syndrome include:

- A stone lodged in the gallbladder neck
- Compression or narrowing of the common hepatic duct
- Dilation of the bile duct proximal to the blockage
- Shrunken gallbladder with thickened walls.

MRCP has advantages over CT in that it lacks exposure to ionizing radiation, avoids contrast injection and its adverse effects, and visualizes biliary tree anatomy in any anatomical plane.

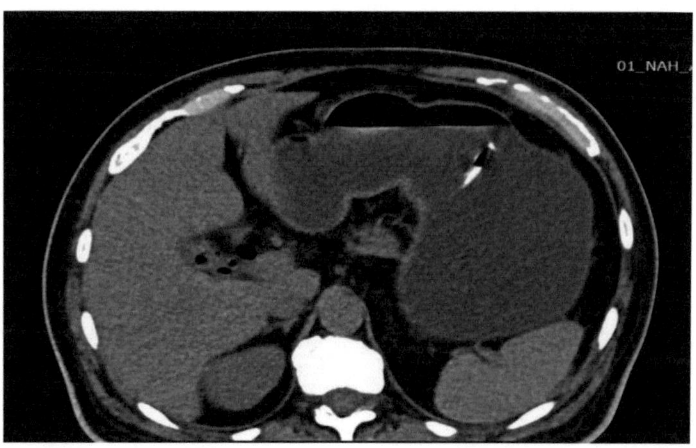

Figure 3.
Contrast-enhanced computed tomography of the abdomen showing pneumobilia with air seen within the gallbladder [24].

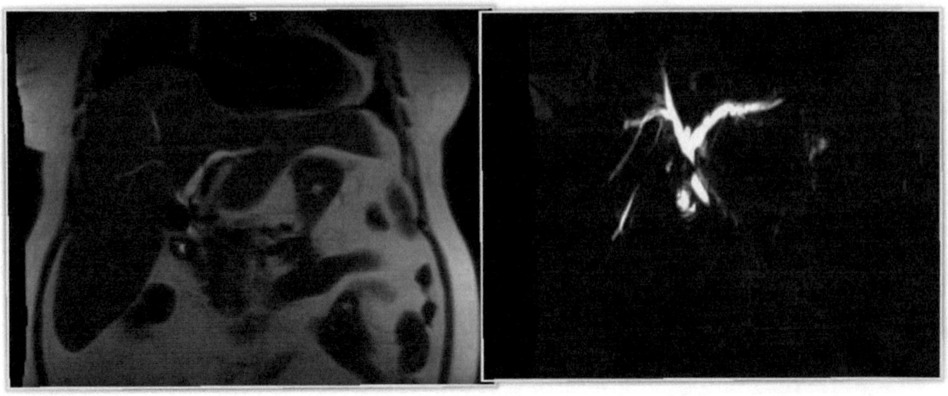

Figure 4.
MRI and MRCP showing stone in cystic duct compressing CHD with mild to moderate IHBRD [24].

Yun et al. evaluated the diagnostic accuracy of MRCP and CT for Mirizzi syndrome and realized that when both modalities were used together, the overall sensitivity was 96% (compared to 42% for CT alone), specificity was 93.5% (versus 98.5% for CT), positive predictive value was 83.5% (CT: 93%), negative predictive value was 98.5% (CT: 83.5%), and accuracy was 94% (CT: 85%) (**Figure 4**) [24].

6.4 Endoscopic retrograde cholangiopancreaticography

Direct cholangiography (Percutaneous Transhepatic Cholangiography or Endoscopic Retrograde Cholangiopancreaticography) is performed, followed by sonography or computed tomography to delineate the extent and shape of biliary duct obstruction. The salient feature of the syndrome is partial obstruction of the common hepatic duct, which can either be due to external compression at the level of the cystic duct or to a partly or completely eroded calculus [21].

ERCP, though invasive, is widely regarded as the most reliable method for diagnosing Mirizzi syndrome. It serves both diagnostic and therapeutic roles, with sensitivity ranging from 50 to 100% and diagnostic accuracy between 55 and 90%. ERCP findings typically reveal an irregular or hollow defect on the side of the common bile duct near the cystic duct or gallbladder neck.

However, ERCP carries risks of complications, including pancreatitis (3.5%), bleeding (1.3%), cholangitis (1%), perforation (0.1–0.6%), and cardiopulmonary issues related to sedation [25].

In patients who are unsuitable for ERCP, have had unsuccessful ERCP attempts, or have altered anatomy due to prior surgeries, percutaneous transhepatic cholangiography (PTC) offers an alternative imaging approach to evaluate the biliary system.

7. Intraoperative diagnosis

Mirizzi syndrome is frequently diagnosed intraoperatively. During surgery, several signs of the condition may be observed, including an inflamed or contracted gallbladder that distorts Calot's triangle, a gallstone lodged in the infundibulum or cystic duct, significant fibrosis in the region, and adhesions beneath the liver. If bile leakage is noted after removing an impacted stone, it strongly suggests the presence of a cholecystobiliary fistula. Intraoperative cholangiography is employed to determine the size and location of the fistula, identify stones within the bile ducts, evaluate the condition of the bile ducts, and remove any residual stones post-surgery. However, this is technically challenging and has a high chance of bile duct injury since anatomical distortions are often seen in Calot's triangle [26].

8. Treatment

Surgical management is the preferred method of managing Mirizzi syndrome, but it is very challenging, as extensive adhesions resulting from chronic inflammation, along with the development of cholecystobiliary or cholecystoenteric fistulas, can significantly distort the anatomy. These changes heighten the risk of common bile duct (CBD) injury or may lead to hemorrhage during the dissection around Calot's triangle.

8.1 Open technique

Traditionally, open cholecystectomy has been the treatment of choice for Mirizzi syndrome. In type I Mirizzi syndrome cases, removal of the gallbladder completely is usually feasible, and it may also be possible for types II and III Mirizzi syndrome, based on the severity of inflammation and anatomical distortions in Calot's triangle. An alternative approach, i.e., the fundus-first approach, is recommended, where the dissection begins at the gallbladder's fundus and moves toward Hartmann's pouch. In cases with significant adhesions in Calot's triangle, subtotal cholecystectomy is a safer and more practical alternative [27].

Choledochoplasty is a surgical method employed after subtotal cholecystectomy, where the remaining portion of the gallbladder or cystic duct is used to repair a cholecysto-choledochal fistula. The repair can be done by primary closure or by utilizing the cuff of the gallbladder for reconstruction, with or without inserting a T-tube into the common bile duct (CBD). This technique is generally applied for type II Mirizzi syndrome and selected cases of type III [28].

When a cholecystobiliary fistula (Mirizzi syndrome type II or higher) is identified, surgeons typically explore the CBD by either open or laparoscopic techniques. This step is crucial; stones are present in the CBD in 25–40% of Mirizzi syndrome cases. The bile duct is accessed through a separate incision over the CHD or CBD, and a T-tube drain is placed to safeguard the sutured area. If there is uncertainty about the durability of the tissue repair, the T-tube helps decompress the bile duct, preserves its structure, and reduces the chance of bile leakage. It also enables cholangiography during surgery and offers a pathway for later removal of any remaining stones.

For Mirizzi syndrome type IV, the standard treatment involves cholecystectomy along with removal of the bile duct and reconstruction via hepaticojejunostomy. Some specialists also suggest this approach, including hepaticojejunostomy, is the best option for type III cases [26].

Surgical management of type Vb (gallstone ileus) offers two options: a one-stage procedure, which involves cholecystectomy along with fistula repair and stone extraction, and a two-stage procedure, where stone extraction is performed first, followed by cholecystectomy and fistula repair at a later time. The two-stage approach poses risks for the patient, including cholecystitis, cholangitis, and GB malignancy due to the ongoing cholecysto-intestinal fistula. However, it is often recommended for high-risk patients with multiple comorbidities, shock, or significant intra-abdominal inflammation or adhesions [17].

8.2 Laparoscopic technique

Initially, this technique was regarded as an absolute contraindication for treating Mirizzi syndrome. Key reasons included a sessile gallbladder, severe adhesions in Calot's triangle, the reliance on the fundus-first approach, the frequent presence of bilio-enteric fistulas, and the need to rule out malignancy [12].

However, with advancements in laparoscopic methods and technology, this approach is now becoming a viable option for managing more complex cases of Mirizzi syndrome, provided the surgeon possesses adequate expertise and patients are carefully chosen. Yetisir et al. reported a successful case of laparoscopic subtotal cholecystectomy and cholecysto-colic fistula resection in a patient with type Va Mirizzi syndrome, using the Tri-Staple device. The patient recovered well and without any symptoms at a follow-up of 8 months [28]. In a recent study, Gomez et al. reported the successful use of laparoscopic cholecystectomy combined with fistula resection and primary closure in 16 patients diagnosed with type Va Mirizzi syndrome [29].

A safe and effective approach for managing Mirizzi syndrome is laparoscopic transfistulous bile duct exploration. Chuang et al. [30] introduced this technique in 2016, which involves initiating dissection from the fundus, performing an infundibulotomy to access the impacted stone and fistula, and conducting a subtotal cholecystectomy. This method has been primarily applied to cases of type II and IV Mirizzi syndrome.

Senra et al. employed an infundibulotomy approach to reach the common bile duct (CBD) with choledochoscopy in patients with type II or higher Mirizzi syndrome, avoiding the need for fistulotomy or choledochotomy. This method eliminated the requirement for obtaining a critical view of safety, thereby reducing the risks associated with dissection in Calot's triangle [31].

Laser-assisted bile duct exploration using the laparoendoscopy (LABEL) approach is a new technique that is preferred for large stones. The LABEL technique enables the fragmentation of big impacted CBD stones into fine pieces, simplifying stone removal during laparoscopic CBD exploration and reducing the need for choledochotomy [32].

8.3 Robot-assisted techniques

Recently, researchers have highlighted the benefits of robot-assisted approaches for treating Mirizzi syndrome. Unlike laparoscopy, robotic systems provide superior visualization through a 3D camera with depth perception, enabling surgeons to execute precise tissue manipulation and intracorporeal suturing using endowrist instruments. Additionally, this approach minimizes the need for partial cholecystectomy, reducing related complications while effectively addressing cholecystobiliary fistulas. Combining this technique with endoscopic methods can further improve treatment outcomes [33].

Mirizzi syndrome can be successfully managed using a minimally invasive technique that integrates robot-assisted surgery with planned preoperative and postoperative ERCP. The treatment approach includes a preoperative ERCP for precise diagnosis and placement of an endoscopic stent. Robotic surgery is then utilized for gallbladder removal and repair of the defect in the common duct. Finally, a postoperative ERCP is conducted to remove the stent. This strategy offers the advantages of minimally invasive surgery for this complex gallbladder condition, such as avoidance of T-tube insertion, reduced hospital stay, smaller incisions, improved cosmetic outcomes, potentially lower blood loss, and fewer postoperative complications [34].

8.4 Intraoperative imaging

Intraoperative cholangiography (IOC) is a valuable tool for assessing the size and position of a cholecystobiliary fistula, detecting bile duct stones, and evaluating the bile duct wall. It also assists in the removal of any remaining stones post-surgery. However, performing IOC can be technically challenging due to anatomical alterations in Calot's triangle, which may increase the risk of bile duct injury [35].

Laparoscopic ultrasonography offers real-time, multi-angle imaging of the bile ducts. It is particularly valuable when Mirizzi syndrome has not been identified before surgery or when it is suspected during the procedure [4].

Near-infrared fluorescence cholangiography with indocyanine green (ICG) dye is a newer technique used during laparoscopic cholecystectomy to enhance bile duct visibility. This method effectively improves the identification of extrahepatic biliary structures, such as the common hepatic and common bile ducts. Compared to intraoperative cholangiography, it offers advantages like shorter procedure times, no need for cystic duct cannulation, and the absence of radiation exposure [36].

These intraoperative imaging techniques are helpful in defining biliary anatomy, especially when Calot's triangle is frozen and there is anomalous anatomy. They also improve the success rate of stone removal from the common bile duct and reduce the risk of bile duct injury.

8.5 Role of endoscopic interventions

ERCP can complement surgical treatment, but complete management still requires gallbladder removal through surgery. This technique enables sphincterotomy for stone extraction and supports procedures like stent placement or naso-biliary tube insertion. It is particularly useful for patients who are not fit for surgery or those who present with acute cholangitis, where decompression of the biliary tract serves as a temporary solution before definitive treatment. Furthermore, ERCP with biliary stent placement can support cholecystectomy or aid in closing a cholecystobiliary fistula by maintaining the patency of the common bile duct. A combined strategy involving ERCP and laparoscopic surgery offers a minimally invasive treatment option for managing Mirizzi syndrome [37]. In addition, cholangioscopy helps to get tissue sampling in some patients to rule out malignancy.

9. Conclusion

Over time, the understanding and treatment of Mirizzi syndrome have significantly advanced. In spite of the availability of advanced diagnostic tools, this condition is frequently identified during surgery. Treating Mirizzi syndrome can be complex, especially for surgeons with limited experience, and necessitates a tailored approach depending on the surgeon's expertise and available resources. Collaboration with a multidisciplinary team is crucial to ensure optimal long-term outcomes. Even for experienced surgeons, having contingency plans, like subtotal cholecystectomy, is recommended when the surgical conditions become challenging.

Author details

Karamveer Singh*, Arunkumar V, Amit Gupta, Satish Ammapalem and Monisha Selvarasu
Department of Surgery, All India Institute of Medical Science, Rishikesh, India

*Address all correspondence to: singhkaramveer28@gmail.com

References

[1] Koo JGA, Tham HY, Toh EQ, Chia C, Thien A, Shelat VG. Mirizzi syndrome-the past, present, and future. Medicina (Kaunas, Lithuania). 2023;**60**(1):12

[2] Shirah BH, Shirah HA, Albeladi KB. Mirizzi syndrome: Necessity for safe approach in dealing with diagnostic and treatment challenges. Annals of Hepato-Biliary-Pancreatic Surgery. 2017;**21**(3):122-130

[3] Chen H, Siwo EA, Khu M, Tian Y. Current trends in the management of Mirizzi syndrome: A review of literature. Medicine (Baltimore). 2018;**97**(4):e9691

[4] Valderrama-Treviño AI, Granados-Romero JJ, Espejel-Deloiza M, Chernitzky-Camaño J, Barrera Mera B, Estrada-Mata AG, et al. Updates in Mirizzi syndrome. Hepatobiliary Surgery and Nutrition. 2017;**6**(3):170-178

[5] Beltrán MA. Mirizzi syndrome: History, current knowledge and proposal of a simplified classification. World Journal of Gastroenterology: WJG. 2012;**18**(34):4639-4650

[6] Abou-Saif A, Al-Kawas FH. Complications of gallstone disease: Mirizzi syndrome, cholecystocholedochal fistula, and gallstone ileus. The American Journal of Gastroenterology. 2002;**97**(2):249-254

[7] Beltran MA, Csendes A. Mirizzi syndrome and gallstone ileus: An unusual presentation of gallstone disease. Journal of Gastrointestinal Surgery: Official Journal of the Society for Surgery of the Alimentary Tract. 2005;**9**(5):686-689

[8] Pemberton M, Wells AD. The Mirizzi syndrome. Postgraduate Medical Journal. 1997;**73**(862):487-490

[9] Yip AW, Chow WC, Chan J, Lam KH. Mirizzi syndrome with cholecystocholedochal fistula: Preoperative diagnosis and management. Surgery. 1992;**111**(3):335-338

[10] Klekowski J, Piekarska A, Góral M, Kozula M, Chabowski M. The current approach to the diagnosis and classification of Mirizzi syndrome. Diagnostics (Basel). 2021;**11**(9):1660. DOI: 10.3390/diagnostics11091660

[11] Csendes A, Diaz JC, Burdiles P, Maluenda F, Nava O. Mirizzi syndrome and cholecystobiliary fistula: A unifying classification. The British Journal of Surgery. 1989;**76**(11):1139-1143

[12] Payá-Llorente C, Vázquez-Tarragón A, Alberola-Soler A, Martínez-Pérez A, Martínez-López E, Santarrufina-Martínez S, et al. Mirizzi syndrome: A new insight provided by a novel classification. Annals of Hepato-Biliary-Pancreatic Surgery. 2017;**21**(2):67-75. DOI: 10.14701/ahbps.2017.21.2.67

[13] Ibrarullah M, Mishra T, Das AP. Mirizzi syndrome. The Indian Journal of Surgery. 2008;**70**(6):281-287

[14] Yeh CN, Jan YY, Chen MF. Laparoscopic treatment for Mirizzi syndrome. Surgical Endoscopy. 2003;**17**(10):1573-1578

[15] Curet MJ, Rosendale DE, Congilosi S. Mirizzi syndrome in a native American population. American Journal of Surgery. 1994;**168**(6):616-621

[16] Khokhar I, Adourian M, Delia E, Mohan G, Mathew M. Mirizzi syndrome: A case report and review of the literature. Cureus. 2022;**14**(4):e24375. DOI: 10.7759/cureus.24375

[17] Clavien P-A, Richon J, Burgan S, Rohner A. Gallstone ileus. The British Journal of Surgery. 1990;77:737-742

[18] Gaduputi V, Tariq H, Rahnemai-Azar AA, Dev A, Farkas DT. Gallstone ileus with multiple stones: Where Rigler triad meets Bouveret's syndrome. World Journal of Gastrointestinal Surgery. 2015;7(12):394-397. DOI: 10.4240/wjgs.v7.i12.394

[19] Bhandari TR, Wong JL, Ahmad J, Akbari K, Menon V. Bouveret's syndrome: An old diagnosis. A modern multimodality approach (endoscopic and robotic surgical) of gastric outlet obstruction: Report of two cases. International Journal of Surgery Case Reports. 2024;**114**:109134. DOI: 10.1016/j.ijscr.2023.109134

[20] Moshref LH, Mandili RA, Almaghrabi M, Abdulwahab RA, Alosaimy RA, Miro J. Elevation of CA 19-9 in Mirizzi syndrome in the absence of malignancy: A case report. The American Journal of Case Reports. 2021;**22**:e931819. DOI: 10.12659/AJCR.931819

[21] Becker CD, Hassler H, Terrier F. Preoperative diagnosis of the Mirizzi syndrome: Limitations of sonography and computed tomography. American Journal of Roentgenology: AJR. 1984;**143**(3):591-596. DOI: 10.2214/ajr.143.3.591

[22] Cui Y, Liu Y, Li Z, Zhao E, Zhang H, Cui N. Appraisal of diagnosis and surgical approach for Mirizzi syndrome. ANZ Journal of Surgery. 2012;**82**(10):708-713

[23] Laing FC, Jeffrey RB Jr. Choledocholithiasis and cystic duct obstruction: Difficult ultrasonographic diagnosis. Radiology. 1983;**146**(2):475-479. DOI: 10.1148/radiology.146.2.6849098

[24] Yun EJ, Choi CS, Yoon DY, Seo YL, Chang SK, Kim JS, et al. Combination of magnetic resonance cholangiopancreatography and computed tomography for preoperative diagnosis of the Mirizzi syndrome. Radiography. Aug 2009;**15**(3):236-240

[25] Yonetci N, Kutluana U, Yilmaz M, Sungurtekin U, Tekin K. The incidence of Mirizzi syndrome in patients undergoing endoscopic retrograde cholangiopancreatography. Hepatobiliary & Pancreatic Diseases International. 2008;**7**(5):520-524

[26] Safioleas M, Stamatakos M, Safioleas P, Smyrnis A, Revenas C, Safioleas C. Mirizzi syndrome: An unexpected problem of cholelithiasis. Our experience with 27 cases. International Seminars in Surgical Oncology. 2008;**5**:12. DOI: 10.1186/1477-7800-5-12

[27] Xu X, Hong T, Li B, Liu W, He X, Zheng C. Mirizzi syndrome: Our experience with 27 cases in PUMC hospital. Chinese Medical Sciences Journal. 2013;**28**(3):172-177

[28] Yetişir F, Şarer AE, Acar HZ, Parlak O, Basaran B, Yazıcıoğlu O. Laparoscopic resection of cholecystocolic fistula and subtotal cholecystectomy by tri-staple in a Type V Mirizzi syndrome. Case Reports in Hepatology. 2016;**2016**:6434507

[29] Gómez D, Pedraza M, Cabrera LF, Mendoza Zuchini A, Arrieta GM, Aparicio BS, et al. Minimally invasive management of Mirizzi syndrome Va: Case series and narrative review of the literature. Cirugia Espanola. 2022;**100**(7):404-409

[30] Chuang SH, Yeh MC, Chang CJ. Laparoscopic transfistulous bile duct exploration for Mirizzi syndrome type II: A simplified standardized technique.

Surgical Endoscopy. 2016;**30**(12):5635-5646. DOI: 10.1007/s00464-016-4911-0

[31] Senra F, Navaratne L, Acosta A, Martínez-Isla A. Laparoscopic management of type II Mirizzi syndrome. Surgical Endoscopy. 2020;**34**(5):2303-2312. DOI: 10.1007/s00464-019-07316-6

[32] Navarro-Sánchez A, Ashrafian H, Segura-Sampedro JJ, Martínez-Isla A. LABEL procedure: Laser-assisted bile duct exploration by laparoendoscopy for choledocholithiasis: Improving surgical outcomes and reducing technical failure. Surgical Endoscopy. 2017;**31**(5):2103-2108. DOI: 10.1007/s00464-016-5206-1

[33] Magge D, Steve J, Novak S, Slivka A, Hogg M, Zureikat A, et al. Performing the difficult cholecystectomy using combined endoscopic and robotic techniques: How I do it. Journal of Gastrointestinal Surgery: Official Journal of the Society for Surgery of the Alimentary Tract. 2017;**21**(3):583-589

[34] Lee KF, Chong CN, Ma KW, Cheung E, Wong J, Cheung S, et al. A minimally invasive strategy for Mirizzi syndrome: The combined endoscopic and robotic approach. Surgical Endoscopy. 2014;**28**(9):2690-2694. DOI: 10.1007/s00464-014-3529-3

[35] Lai EC, Lau WY. Mirizzi syndrome: History, present and future development. ANZ Journal of Surgery. 2006;**76**(4):251-257. DOI: 10.1111/j.1445-2197.2006.03690.x

[36] Wang C, Peng W, Yang J, Li Y, Yang J, Hu X, et al. Application of near-infrared fluorescent cholangiography using indocyanine green in laparoscopic cholecystectomy. The Journal of International Medical Research. 2020;**48**(12):300060520979224. DOI: 10.1177/0300060520979224

[37] Li B, Li X, Zhou WC, He MY, Meng WB, Zhang L, et al. Effect of endoscopic retrograde cholangiopancreatography combined with laparoscopy and choledochoscopy on the treatment of Mirizzi syndrome. Chinese Medical Journal. 2013;**126**(18):3515-3518

Chapter 6

Gallbladder Carcinoma: A Comprehensive Review and Recent Updates

Amit Gupta, Ammapalem Satish, Karamveer Singh, Arunkumar V and Prasoon Saxena

Abstract

Gallbladder cancer is the most common biliary tract cancer. It predominantly affects females, individuals of advanced age, and those with chronic gallbladder inflammation, gallstones, or infections. It is often diagnosed at an advanced stage due to its indolent early course and aggressive nature, leading to poor prognosis. The global incidence varies significantly, with high rates in Chile, India, and Pakistan. Risk factors include chronic inflammation, gallstones, polyps, porcelain gallbladder, primary sclerosing cholangitis, and genetic mutations. Diagnosis relies on imaging modalities such as ultrasound, computed tomography (CT), magnetic resonance imaging (MRI), and tumor markers (CEA, CA 19–9). Gallbladder Reporting and Data System (GB-RADS) aids in risk assessment. Staging follows the American Joint Committee on Cancer (AJCC) 8th edition criteria, which emphasize tumor location and lymph node involvement. Surgical resection remains the only curative approach. Staging laparoscopy helps avoid unnecessary surgeries in metastatic disease. Adjuvant chemotherapy [e.g., capecitabine] and immunotherapy [durvalumab, pembrolizumab] improve survival outcomes. Despite advancements, survival remains poor, particularly in late-stage disease, underscoring the need for early detection, minimally invasive techniques, and novel therapeutic strategies. Ongoing trials continue to refine treatment protocols for improved prognosis.

Keywords: gallbladder cancer, gallstones, radical cholecystectomy, porcelain gallbladder, primary sclerosing cholangitis, GB-RADS, gallbladder polyp

1. Introduction

Gallbladder cancer (GBC) is the most common biliary tract cancer and fifth among GI malignancies. It is linked to risk factors like female gender, advanced age, gallstones, and chronic infections with high incidence in regions like India and South America. Gallbladder cancer is often detected at a late stage due to its lack of early symptoms and aggressive tendency to spread quickly. Diagnosis involves CT, MRI, and pathological staging. Prognosis depends on stage, with early-stage survival at 76.6% and advanced-stage at 2.2%. Early detection and aggressive surgical approach are warranted [1].

Advances in diagnostics, minimally invasive surgery, and systemic treatments like targeted therapy and immunotherapy are of paramount importance.

2. Incidence

The overall incidence of GBC worldwide is estimated to be 1–2 cases per 100,000 people per year. Incidence varies globally, with higher incidence observed in certain geographic regions such as South America (16–27/100000 in females and 8–12/100000 in males) and parts of Asia [particularly India—22/100000, Pakistan—11/100000, and Japan—7/100000]. It is the most common cause of

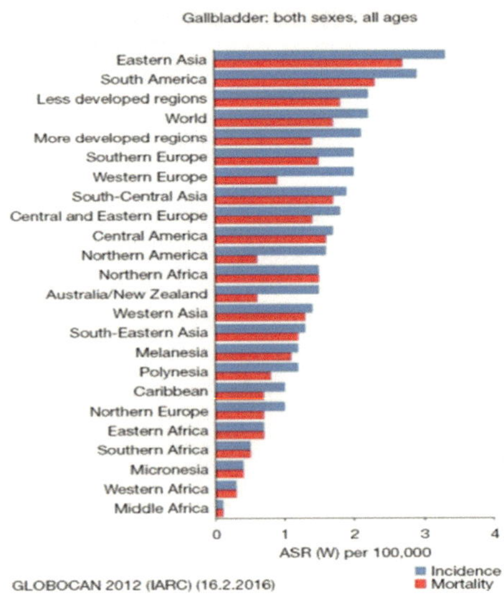

Figure 1.
Showing geographical variation in incidence as highlighted in global studies [5].

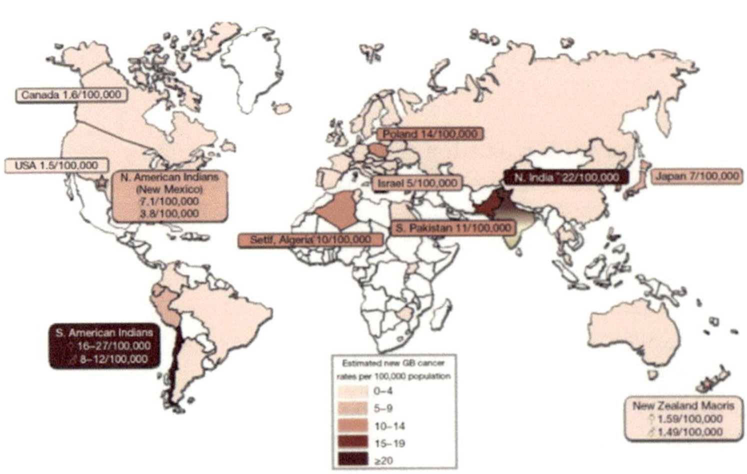

Figure 2.
Showing age-standardized rates of GBC [6].

cancer-related deaths among Chilean women (27 cases/100000/year), surpassing even cervical and breast cancer [2, 3]. It is relatively rare in Western countries. Other high-risk areas include southern Pakistan, northern India, and Eastern Europe [4]. Israel and Japan have intermediate incidences (**Figures 1** and **2**) [7].

3. Risk factors

Chronic inflammation of the gallbladder is the primary pathogenic mechanism linked to gallbladder carcinoma [8].

1. Age; Advanced age is a major risk factor for gallbladder cancer, with the typical age of diagnosis between 50 and 55 years. In India, however, the disease tends to present a decade earlier [9].

2. Gender; Women have a 2 to 6 times higher risk of developing GBC. Estrogen increases cholesterol saturation in bile, leading to higher gallstone formation, a major risk factor for GBC. Progesterone reduces gallbladder motility, causing bile stasis and an increased risk of chronic inflammation further contributing to the development of gallbladder cancer [10].

3. Gallstones; Presence of gallstone disease is the most common condition associated with GBC. Around 45–60% of GBC cases had a history of cholelithiasis [9, 11]. Several studies suggest that size of the gallstone size and GBC are directly related with larger stones greater than 3 cm being associated with a 10 times greater risk of GBC. The presence of multiple gallstones and increased duration are also associated with an increased risk of GBC.

4. Premalignant conditions

1. Porcelain GB:- It is associated with a high risk for gallbladder cancer. Older studies reported a 21% incidence of gallbladder cancer leading to the recommendation of prophylactic cholecystectomy [12]. Recent studies suggest a lower cancer risk (around 6%), but focal calcification has a higher risk compared to diffuse calcification which carries a lower risk but warrants surveillance.

2. Polyps: GB polyps can be either pseudo polyps as is the case in cholesterol polyps or true GB polyps which may be benign or malignant. Polyps are usually asymptomatic. Large, sessile, or solitary polyps, the presence of gallstones, older age, and rapid growth are indicators of a polyp's malignant potential [13].

3. Primary sclerosing cholangitis (PSC); It is a chronic, progressive liver disease characterized by chronic inflammation and scarring (fibrosis) of the bile ducts, and bile stasis, leading to a risk of developing GBC [14]. The estimated lifetime incidence of GBC is from 3–14% [15].

5. Etiopathogenesis

GBC is a multifactorial disease with complex interaction between genetic and environmental factors. Chronic cholecystitis, caused by recurrent infections and inflammation of the gallbladder mucosa due to gallstones, triggers the release of inflammatory mediators. Epithelial damage and repair in repeated cycles lead to metaplasia which eventually progresses to dysplasia. Over time, dysplasia can develop in-situ and then invasive carcinoma. This process typically takes around 15 years. Studies indicate that the average age of patients with dysplasia, early malignancy, advanced malignancy, and metastasis is 46.3, 57.5, 59.0, and 61.1 years respectively, for metastatic cancer [8]. Gallstones and PSC can lead to H.pylori infection and chronic cholecystitis [16, 17]. Mutations in the P53 gene are implicated in the development of GBC [18]. Alterations in the NLRP3 gene leading to mutations in Interleukin-10/1β, TNF-α, and COX-2 genes contribute to the development of GBC.

Several metals like arsenic, boron, lithium, and molybdenum were implicated in the pathogenesis of gallstone and GBC. Arsenic has a carcinogenic effect due to DNA damage and genomic alterations [19].

The apoptosis pathway triggered by TNF-R1 and other death receptors, including TRAIL, FAS, and CD-95, leads to sequential activation of procaspase-8 and Phospholipase A2.

6. Pathways of lymphatic spread in gallbladder cancer

The lymphatic drainage of the gallbladder is via multiple pathways [20].

1. The principal pathway of spread is cholecysto-retropancreatic pathway which drains along cystic nodes, pericholedochal nodes (station 12b), portocaval node (station 12p), and superior retro pancreatic node (station 13) to paraaortic nodes (station 16).

2. The cholecysto-celiac pathway, the next most common pathway, drains along cystic nodes and medially along the hepatoduodenal ligament (station 12a)

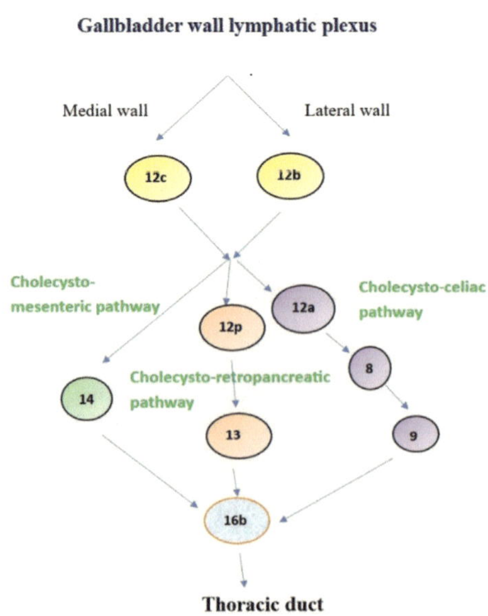

Figure 3.
Pathways of lymphatic spread in GBC.

superior to the head of the pancreas to the portal vein (station 12), hepatic artery (station 8), and celiac axis (station 9).

3. The cholecysto-mesenteric pathway drains to the left in front of the portal vein (station 12) connecting with the nodes at the root of the mesentery (superior mesenteric nodes, station 14).

4. A hilar route that ascends directly towards the hepatic hilum has been described in an animal model (**Figure 3**).

7. Clinical presentation

Gallbladder cancer (GBC) often presents late due to its nonspecific symptoms leading to delayed diagnosis and poor prognosis. In the early stages, it may remain asymptomatic or mimic benign gallbladder diseases such as cholelithiasis or cholecystitis. As the disease progresses, patients commonly experience persistent right upper quadrant (RUQ) abdominal pain, which may radiate to the back. Unintended weight loss, anorexia, and fatigue are common systemic symptoms indicating advanced disease. Jaundice, resulting from biliary obstruction due to tumor infiltration or compression of the bile ducts, is seen in later stages. Palpable mass in the right upper quadrant may be detected, especially in locally advanced cases. GBC is often incidentally detected during cholecystectomy for suspected benign disease or upon pathological examination. Due to its aggressive nature and vague symptoms, early detection requires a high index of suspicion, particularly in high-risk individuals.

Jaundice in GBC is linked to a poor prognosis, as it often signifies a more advanced stage of the disease. Jaundice in gallbladder cancer [GBC] can arise from various

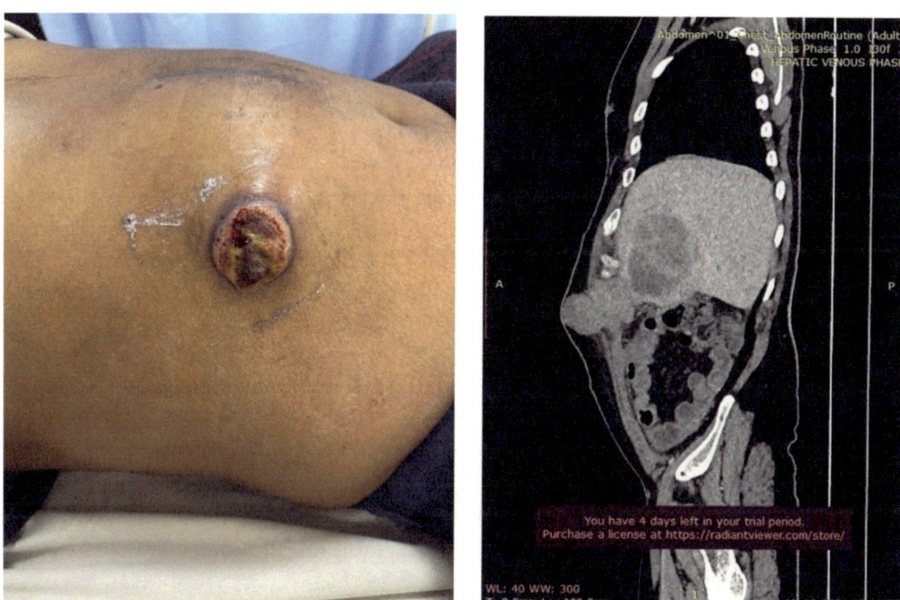

Figure 4.
Patient presented with drain site metastasis with CT showing abdominal wall infiltration.

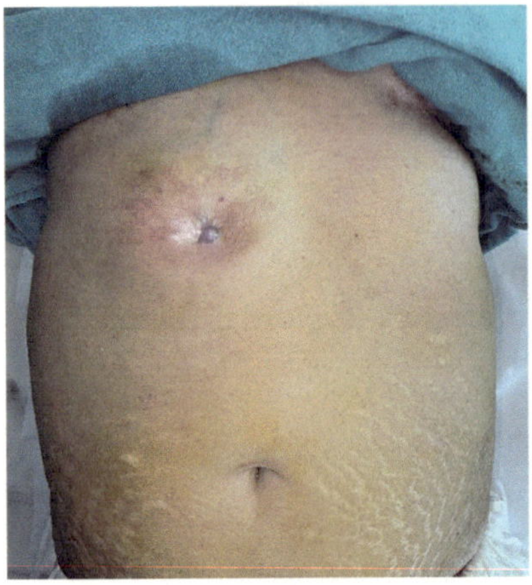

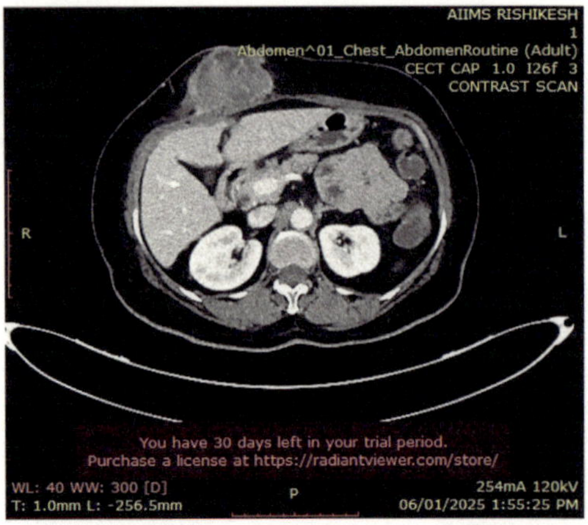

Figure 5.
Patient presented with port site metastasis with CT showing abdominal wall infiltration.

mechanisms, including direct invasion of the CBD by a tumor in the gallbladder neck or cystic duct, leading to mid-CBD obstruction. Tumor infiltration at the hepatic hilum can block the ductal confluence leading to high biliary obstruction. Additionally, tumor extension into the liver parenchyma, particularly in the gallbladder bed, may obstruct the right portal pedicle, resulting in intrahepatic biliary obstruction. Metastatic lymph nodes in the porta hepatis and hepatoduodenal ligament can also compress the CBD at different levels. In some cases, a tumor embolus from a papillary gallbladder tumor can block the CBD.

Furthermore, secondary CBD stones associated with gallstones may contribute to biliary obstruction. These diverse pathways illustrate how GBC can lead to jaundice, influencing disease progression and management (**Figures 4** and 5).

8. Diagnostic workup

8.1 Radiology

Ultrasound is the first-line imaging modality, with findings such as asymmetrical focal thickening of the gallbladder wall or a heterogeneous lesion raising suspicion for malignancy. The GB-RADS has been proposed to stratify cancer risk and guide further imaging decisions. For a more comprehensive assessment, contrast-enhanced CT and/or MRI is recommended. These modalities help evaluate lymph node involvement, distant metastases, direct invasion of adjacent organs, and major vascular invasion [21]. CT cholangiography plays a crucial role in assessing this condition by providing detailed visualization of bile duct dilatation and accurately identifying the level of obstruction. It helps differentiate between benign and malignant biliary strictures, allowing for more precise diagnosis and treatment planning. CT findings in gallbladder cancer typically include a heterogeneous but predominantly hypodense mass in the gallbladder, with or without liver involvement in around 60% of cases. Gallbladder wall thickening is observed in 20–30% characterized by focal, asymmetrical, and irregular patterns, distinguishing it from the diffuse, symmetrical, and uniform thickening seen in benign disease. An intraluminal polypoidal mass is present in 15–25% of cases (**Figure 6**).

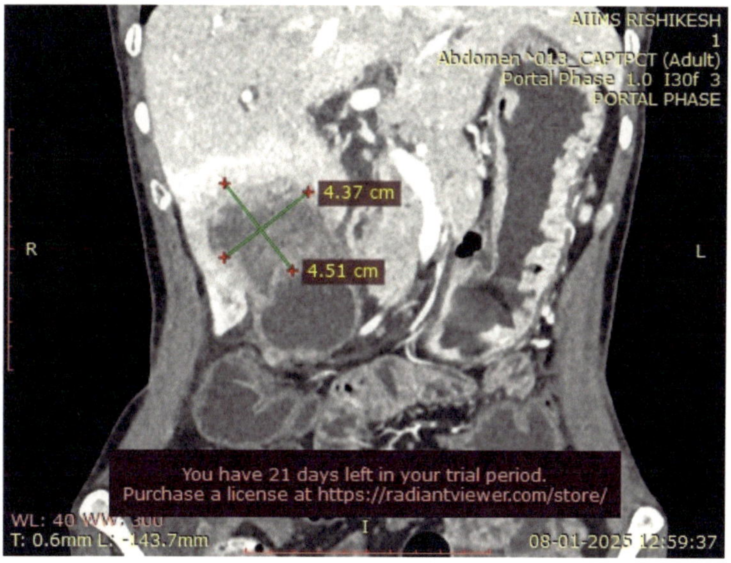

Figure 6.
CT scan showing gallbladder mass infiltrating segment 4b and 5.

For patients with jaundice, additional evaluation with cholangiography is necessary to assess hepatic and biliary tumor invasion, with MRCP preferred over ERCP. Dynamic MRI is considered a valuable tool for staging advanced gallbladder carcinoma. MRI combined with MRCP is highly sensitive in detecting obstructive jaundice, liver invasion, and lymph node metastases. Reported sensitivity rates for detecting direct hepatic invasion and lymph node involvement on MRI can reach up to 100% and 92%, respectively [22].

8.2 GB-RADS

GB-RADS is an ultrasound-based risk stratification tool designed to enhance consistency in interpreting, reporting, and assessing the malignancy risk of gallbladder wall thickening in non-acute settings. The system categorizes findings into six levels [GB-RADS 0–5], with each level representing a progressively higher risk of GBC. Components include wall involvement [focal vs. circumferential], the presence of a layered appearance, interface between the gallbladder and liver, and intramural characteristics such as cysts or echogenic foci [23]. High-risk findings, such as polyps >1 cm, focal irregular thickening, or mass-like lesions, raise suspicion for malignancy and often warrant early surgical intervention. It enhances early cancer detection, reduces unnecessary surgeries, and improves clinical decision-making for better patient outcomes (**Figures 7–9**).

8.3 Tumor markers

CEA (Normal value <5 ng/ml), CA 19–9 (Normal value <37 U/ml), and CA-125 (Normal value <35 U/ml) testing are included in the initial workup for gallbladder cancer alongside imaging studies. Elevated levels of these markers may indicate malignancy, with CA 19–9 demonstrating higher specificity but lower sensitivity [15]. Very high CA 19–9 levels (>1000 U/mL) are strongly correlated with poor prognosis

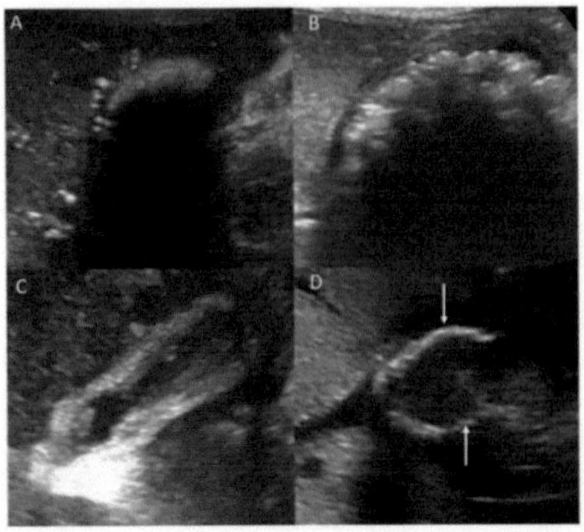

Figure 7.
GB-RADS 0 (inadequate evaluation). A and B. Wall-echoshadow complex. C. Contracted gallbladder. D. Porcelain gallbladder.

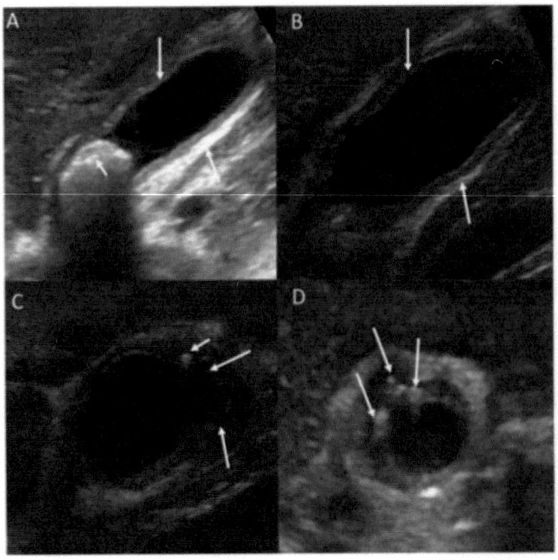

Figure 8.
GB-RADS 2 (benign). A and B. Symmetric circumferential mural thickening with layered appearance. Note that the inner and outer hyperechoic layers are distinctly seen in both A and B (arrows). There is a calculus in the lumen in a (short arrow). C and D. Focal thickening with intramural changes. There are intramural cysts (arrows) and echogenic focus (short arrow) in C. Note the multiple intramural echogenic foci in D (arrows).

and widespread metastasis. CA 19–9 can be elevated in other malignancies or in cases of jaundice from non-cancerous causes. CEA is not specific to gallbladder cancer. High preoperative CEA levels are linked to poor prognosis and higher recurrence rates. Rising CEA levels post-surgery or during chemotherapy may indicate disease progression or recurrence. CA 242 (marker for hepatic infiltration), when combined with other tumor markers like CA 19–9 and CEA, enhances diagnostic accuracy for GBC. NCCN recommends these tests for baseline assessment rather than as definitive diagnostic tools.

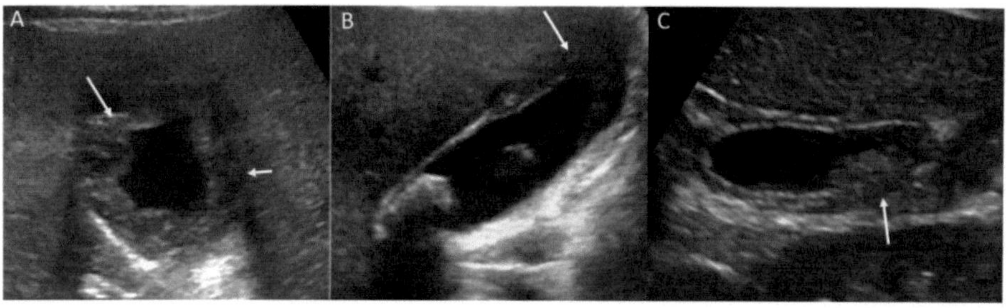

Figure 9.
GB-RADS 4 (malignancy is likely). A. Asymmetric circumferential mural thickening (arrow) without layered appearance and with loss of interface with liver (short arrow). B. Focal thickening in the fundus with no intramural features and loss of interface with liver (arrow). C. Focal thickening with no intramural features along the peritoneal aspect (arrow).

8.4 Molecular markers

Biochemical and molecular markers play a crucial role in the early detection, prognosis, and targeted therapy of GBC. Molecular markers have provided deeper insights into the pathogenesis of GBC, with mutations in KRAS, TP53, IDH1/2, and PIK3CA frequently observed. Overexpression of HER2/neu has been identified in a subset of patients, making HER2-targeted therapies a potential treatment avenue. Additionally, alterations in FGFR2 and BRAF pathways have opened possibilities for precision medicine approaches. Epigenetic changes, including aberrant DNA methylation and microRNA dysregulation, also contribute to tumor progression and may serve as future therapeutic targets. The integration of these biomarkers into clinical practice holds promise for improving early diagnosis, risk stratification, and personalized treatment strategies in gallbladder cancer.

Platelet distribution width [PDW] has high sensitivity [90%] and specificity [95%] in identifying GBC and is considered a cost-effective marker [24]. In a study by Gupta A et al., Red cell Distribution Width (RDW) can be used as a surrogate biomarker to predict tumor stage and tumor burden in GBC [25]. In a study by Rishit Mani et al., GBC had 16% expression of HER2 with a significant degree of differentiation with ER and PR having no significant expression in GBC [26]. A prospective observational study [2017–2020] including fifty newly diagnosed cases shows the expression of molecular markers survivin, COX-2, Her2 neu, p53, and p16in GBC (**Table 1**) [27].

8.5 Changes in AJCC 8th edition

T2 category was subdivided into T2a for peritoneal side and T2b for hepatic side, as tumors of later were believed to have poorer prognoses. The N classification transitioned from a location-based system (7th edition) to a numerical approach, categorizing lymph node metastases as N1 with 1 to 3 nodes and N2 with ≥4 nodes. Additionally, the new guidelines recommend examining at least six lymph nodes for accurate staging. Stage groupings were also revised, introducing Stage IIA [T2aN0M0] and Stage IIB [T2bN0M0]. While the changes in the N category enhanced prognostic accuracy, studies suggest that distinguishing between T2a and T2b may not significantly affect survival stratification [28].

Marker type	Examples	Role in GBC	Clinical significance
Serum tumor markers	CA 19–9, CEA	Used for diagnosis and monitoring	Lack specificity; elevated in other biliary diseases
Genetic mutations	KRAS, TP53, IDH1/2, PIK3CA	Common mutations involved in GBC pathogenesis	Potential targets for precision medicine
HER2/neu overexpression	HER2/neu	Present in a subset of GBC cases	Targeted therapy with HER2 inhibitors possible
Signaling pathway alterations	FGFR2, BRAF	Associated with tumor growth and progression	Potential for targeted treatments
Epigenetic changes	DNA methylation, microRNA dysregulation	Contribute to tumor progression	Emerging as potential biomarkers and therapeutic targets

Table 1.
Biochemical and molecular markers in gallbladder cancer, highlighting their role and clinical significance in diagnosis, prognosis, and treatment strategies.

9. Management

9.1 Surgical management

The only potential curative treatment for GBC is surgical resection with negative margins [29]. For T1a tumors, cholecystectomy will suffice, offering nearly 100% long-term survival [30]. However, optimal surgical management for T2 or more advanced tumors is radical cholecystectomy defined as en bloc removal of gallbladder with segments 4b/5 of liver and hepatoduodenal ligament clearance with aortocaval lymph node sampling [31]. The necessity of radical resection for T1b tumors remains controversial, as there is a risk of discovering residual hepatic or nodal disease upon re-resection. Lymph node dissection should encompass hepatoduodenal ligament, porta hepatis, and retroduodenal regions. In certain cases, extended liver resections [beyond segments 4B and 5] and CBD resection may be required to achieve negative margins.

Empiric major resections of liver and bile duct have been associated with increased morbidity without a clear survival benefit [32]. Studies have shown that bile duct resection does not improve lymph node yield or survival outcomes [33]. The AFS-GBC-2009 study by Fuks et al. reported a 60% postoperative morbidity rate in patients undergoing bile duct resection for incidental gallbladder cancer. Bile duct excision should be reserved for cases with adherent nodal disease, locally invasive tumors, or to achieve cystic duct margin negativity [34]. Lymph node clearance is recommended for gallbladder cancer cases beyond T1a stage. For accurate staging, a minimum of six lymph nodes should be excised (**Figures 10–12**).

10. Role of staging laparoscopy

Staging laparoscopy (SL) is used to assess the extent of gallbladder cancer (GBC) before proceeding with definitive surgery. It helps identify peritoneal and liver metastases that may not be visible on imaging, thereby preventing unnecessary laparotomies in patients with unresectable disease. By allowing direct visualization of the abdominal cavity, SL aids in accurate staging and ensures that only patients with

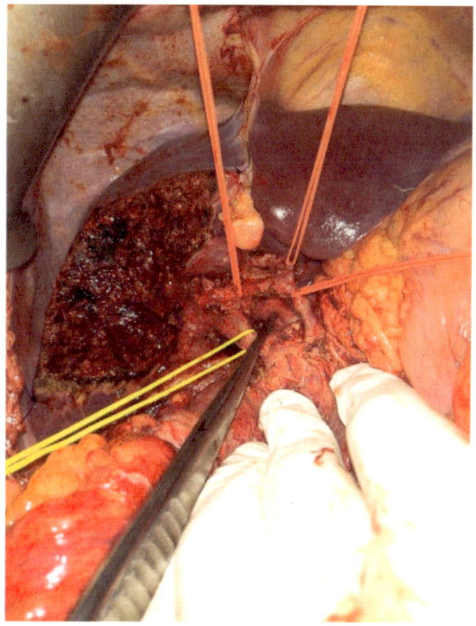

Figure 10.
Post radical cholecystectomy liver bed along with hepatoduodenal ligament clearance showing hepatic artery, portal vein, and bile duct.

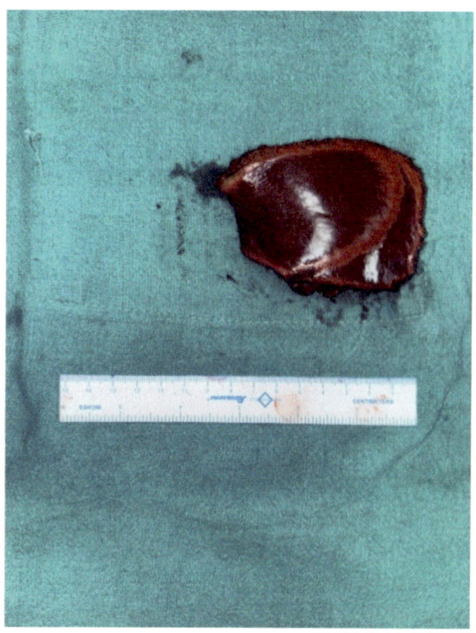

Figure 11.
Incidental GBC (Resected liver specimen).

truly resectable tumors undergo major surgery. It is particularly valuable for patients with suspected advanced disease, as it can detect occult metastases that might alter the treatment plan. In cases where cancer is deemed unresectable, SL allows for early

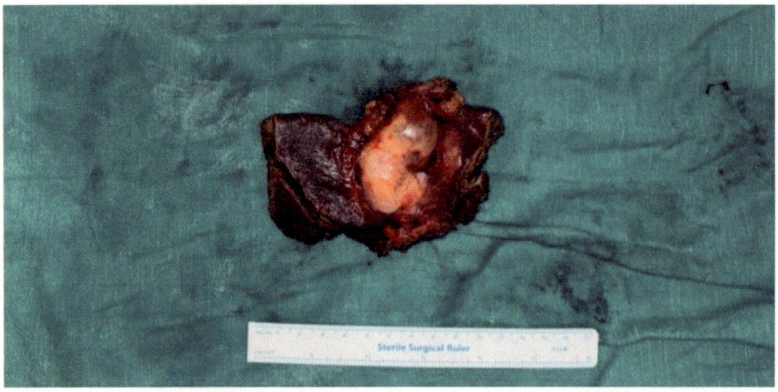

Figure 12.
Gallbladder with resected liver segments (4b/5).

Study	Type	Sample size	Findings
SL in Preventing Nontherapeutic Laparotomies [35]	Prospective	409 patients	SL identified 94.1% of detectable lesions; prevented nontherapeutic laparotomies in 55.9% of unresectable cases and 23.2% of total cases
Two-Stage Laparoscopic Algorithm Study [36]	Prospective Observational	40 patients	Assessed safety and feasibility of a novel two-stage laparoscopic total biopsy method for GBC

Table 2.
Role of staging laparoscopy in gallbladder cancer.

initiation of palliative treatment, avoiding the risks associated with nontherapeutic open surgery. As a result, SL has become an essential tool in the management of gallbladder cancer, improving decision-making and optimizing patient outcomes. Staging laparoscopy is highly effective in detecting metastatic disease or other contra-indications to tumor resection (**Table 2**).

11. Role of minimal invasive surgery in gallbladder cancer

A recent meta-analysis indicates that both laparoscopic and robotic surgery are safe and effective modalities for GBC, with postoperative and survival outcomes comparable to open surgery [OS]. Minimally invasive surgery [MIS] is associated with shorter hospital stays, reduced intraoperative blood loss, and fewer postoperative complications. However, no clear advantage was observed between laparoscopic and robotic approaches [37]. Additionally, fluorescence-guided anatomical resection has been shown to facilitate minimally invasive liver resection with radical lymphadenectomy in selected gallbladder cancer patients.

12. Gallbladder cancer diagnosed after gallbladder surgery [Incidental GBC]

Incidental Gallbladder Carcinoma (IGBC) refers to gallbladder cancer that is unexpectedly detected during or after cholecystectomy for presumed benign

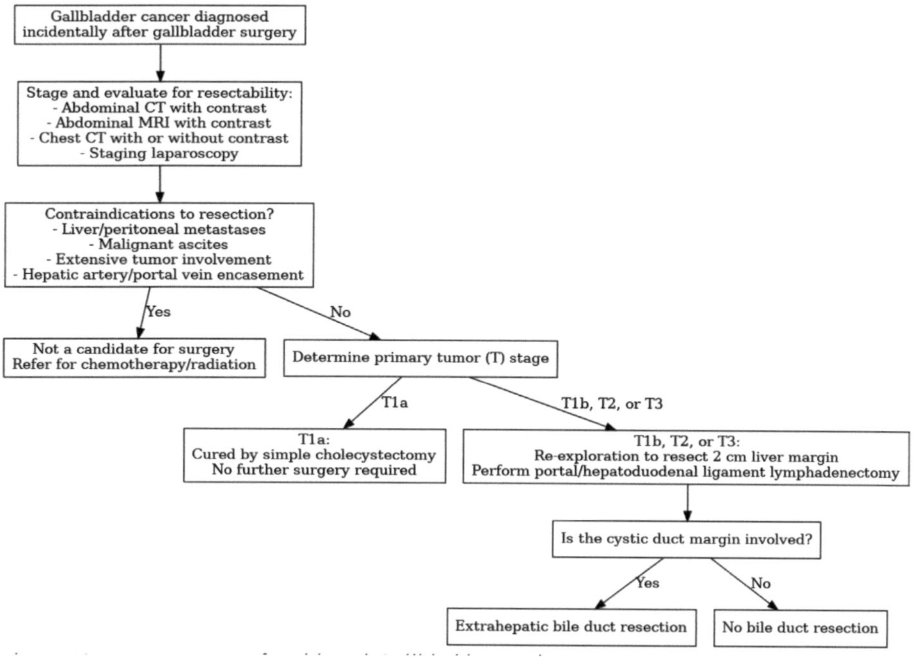

Figure 13.
Management of Incidental Gallbladder carcinoma.

conditions and the diagnosis is typically made on histopathological examination of the removed gallbladder. Incidental GBC was found in 0.25 to 1.5% of patients undergoing laparoscopic cholecystectomy [38]. It is frequently diagnosed post-cholecystectomy and requires stage-based management. Early-stage detection offers a high chance of cure, while advanced cases demand aggressive treatment. Routine histopathological examination of gallbladders, especially in high-risk individuals, is crucial for early diagnosis. Early re-resection, particularly within 6 weeks, may offer survival benefits. Neglected GBC refers to gallbladder cancer that remains undiagnosed or misdiagnosed for an extended period, often due to vague symptoms, lack of early detection, or misinterpretation as benign gallbladder diseases. By the time of diagnosis, the disease is typically advanced (T3/T4) or metastatic (M1), leading to limited treatment options and poor prognosis (**Figure 13**).

13. Unresectable or metastatic disease [Palliation]

Biopsy confirmation is recommended for patients with unresectable or metastatic gallbladder cancer. Unresectable disease includes tumors with distant lymph node metastases in the celiac axis or aortocaval groove, while metastatic disease encompasses distant metastases, nodal involvement beyond the porta hepatis, and extensive porta hepatis involvement leading to jaundice or vascular encasement. Biliary drainage is a suitable palliative intervention and should be considered before resection or systemic therapy if feasible. Palliative options for duodenal obstruction and pain include stenting/naso-jejunal tube placement/gastrojejunostomy and celiac ganglion block, respectively.

14. Adjuvant therapy for localized resected gallbladder cancer

Surgery remains the only curative treatment option for gallbladder cancer [GBC]. However, prognosis remains poor, especially for T3 and/or node-positive disease, due to high rates of recurrence, leading to interest in adjuvant chemotherapy (CT) and radiotherapy (RT). Chemotherapy is commonly used in adjuvant (post-surgery), neoadjuvant (pre-surgery), and palliative settings to improve survival and control disease progression. The standard first-line regimen for advanced GBC is a combination of gemcitabine and cisplatin, which has shown significant survival benefits. An alternative regimen, gemcitabine plus oxaliplatin (GEMOX), is used when cisplatin is contraindicated. In the adjuvant setting, capecitabine-based therapy has been recommended based on the BILCAP trial, which demonstrated improved survival outcomes. Additionally, FOLFOX (5-FU plus oxaliplatin) is considered for refractory cases where gemcitabine-based treatments fail. Support for chemoradiation comes from an analysis of 5029 patients with T1-3N0–1 GBC who underwent surgical resection. This study found that chemoradiation provided the greatest improvement in three-year overall survival compared to chemotherapy alone [39].

15. Neoadjuvant therapy in gallbladder cancer

For patients with good performance status and normal bilirubin levels, the preferred first-line treatment is gemcitabine plus cisplatin, with the addition of immunotherapy [durvalumab or pembrolizumab]. In patients with good performance status but persistent hyperbilirubinemia despite stenting, a fluoropyrimidine plus oxaliplatin regimen, such as capecitabine plus oxaliplatin [CAPOX], is preferred. For those with borderline performance status or significant comorbidities, gemcitabine monotherapy is the recommended treatment.

16. Targetted therapy in gallbladder cancer

Emerging approaches, such as immunotherapy with drugs like durvalumab and pembrolizumab, are being studied in combination with chemotherapy, while targeted therapies like zanidatamab have been approved for HER2-positive gallbladder cancer. As research continues, personalized and targeted therapies are expected to further improve treatment outcomes for gallbladder cancer patients.

Stage	Median survival	5 year survival
Stage 0	>60 months	>90%
Stage 1	45–60 months	60–80%
Stage 2	25–40 months	50–60%
Stage 3	12–24 months	20–40%
Stage 4	4–12 months	<10%

Table 3.
Median survival and five-year survival rates in GBC.

17. Survival and outcomes

The overall five-year survival rate for gallbladder cancer is approximately 20%. However, in patients with localized disease who can undergo surgical resection, five-year survival improves significantly to 65% (**Table 3**).

18. Surveillance

Patients undergoing radical cholecystectomy for gallbladder cancer should be monitored with imaging studies every 3 to 6 months for the first 2 years, followed by every 6 to 12 months for up to 5 years. Additionally, CEA and CA 19–9 levels should be assessed as clinically indicated to aid in detecting recurrence.

19. Screening in gallbladder cancer

Screening for gallbladder cancer (GBC) is not conducted on a population-wide basis due to its low overall incidence and the lack of cost-effective screening tools. However, targeted screening is recommended for high-risk individuals, including those with large gallstones (>3 cm), porcelain gallbladder, gallbladder polyps >1 cm, primary sclerosing cholangitis (PSC), anomalous pancreaticobiliary duct junction (APBDJ), chronic bacterial infections (Salmonella or Helicobacter), and a family history of GBC. In high-risk groups, ultrasound (USG) serves as the first-line screening tool, performed annually to detect gallbladder abnormalities. Although tumor markers like CA 19–9 and CEA lack specificity, they may aid in monitoring disease progression. Emerging biomarkers, including DNA methylation and circulating tumor DNA, are being investigated for early detection. Instead of mass screening, preventive strategies such as early cholecystectomy for high-risk patients, lifestyle modifications, and regular imaging surveillance remain the best approaches to reducing GBC incidence and mortality.

20. Notable trials in gallbladder cancer

Gallbladder cancer poses a challenge in treatment. Over the years, multiple trials investigated chemotherapy to improve patient outcomes, providing insights into the efficacy of chemotherapy, targeted therapy, and immunotherapy. The summary of a few notable trials in gallbladder cancer is given in the following table (**Table 4**).

Trials	Patient population	Treatment arms	Results
BILCAP (2017) [40]	Resected biliary tract cancer	8 cycles of Capecitabine vs. observation (adjuvant)	Capecitabine improved OS (51 vs. 36 months), making it the standard of care for adjuvant therapy.
Prodige 12 (ACCORD 18) (2019) [41]	Resected biliary tract cancers	Adjuvant GEMOX (gemcitabine + oxaliplatin) vs. observation	No significant improvement in relapse-free survival, time to definitive deterioration of quality of life, or overall survival, leading to GEMOX not being recommended for adjuvant therapy

Trials	Patient population	Treatment arms	Results
ABC-02 (2010) [42]	Unresectable/ metastatic biliary tract cancers (including GBC)	Gemcitabine + cisplatin vs. gemcitabine alone	Combination therapy improved OS (11.7 vs. 8.1 months), establishing it as the standard first-line therapy
TOPAZ-1 (2023) [43]	Unresectable/ metastatic biliary tract cancers (25% GBC)	Gemcitabine + cisplatin + durvalumab (immunotherapy)	Adding durvalumab improved progression-free survival and OS, making chemo-immunotherapy a new standard.
Race GB study [44]	Advanced GB malignancy (140 patients)	Consolidation CTRT vs. Observation	consolidation CTRT significantly prolonged overall survival without deterioration in quality of life and should be the alternative standard of care in advanced unresectable GBC.

Table 4.
Notable trials in gallbladder cancer.

Author details

Amit Gupta*, Ammapalem Satish, Karamveer Singh, Arunkumar V and Prasoon Saxena
Department of Surgery, AIIMS, Rishikesh, India

*Address all correspondence to: dramit2411@gmail.com

References

[1] Waller GC, Sarpel U. Gallbladder cancer. Surgical Clinics. 2024;**104**(6):1263-1280

[2] Andia ME, Hsing AW, Andreotti G, Ferreccio C. Geographic variation of gallbladder cancer mortality and risk factors in Chile: A population-based ecologic study. International Journal of Cancer. 2008;**123**:1411-1416

[3] Serra I, Calvo A, Csendes A, Sharp A. Gastric and gallbladder carcinoma in Chile: Epidemiological changes and control programs. Revista Médica de Chile. 1989;**117**:834-836

[4] Randi G, Franceschi S, La Vecchia C. Gallbladder cancer worldwide: Geographical distribution and risk factors. International Journal of Cancer. 2006;**118**:1591-1602

[5] Huang J, Patel HK, Boakye D, Chandrasekar VT, Koulaouzidis A, Lucero-Prisno DE III, et al. Worldwide distribution, associated factors, and trends of gallbladder cancer: A global country-level analysis. Cancer Letters. 2021;**28**(521):238-251

[6] Hundal R, Shaffer EA. Gallbladder cancer: Epidemiology and outcome. Clinical Epidemiology. 2014;**7**:99-109

[7] Lazcano-Ponce EC, Miquel JF, Muñoz N, et al. Epidemiology and molecular pathology of gallbladder cancer. CA: a Cancer Journal for Clinicians. 2001;**51**:349-364

[8] Roa I, Araya JC, Villaseca M, De Aretxabala X, Riedemann P, Endoh K, et al. Preneoplastic lesions and gallbladder cancer: An estimate of the period required for progression. Gastroenterology. 1996;**111**(1):232-236

[9] Dutta U, Bush N, Kalsi D, Popli P, Kapoor VK. Epidemiology of gallbladder cancer in India. Chinese Clinical Oncology. 2019;**8**(4):33

[10] Chen A, Huminer D. The role of estrogen receptors in the development of gallstones and gallbladder cancer. Medical Hypotheses. 1991;**36**(3):259-260

[11] Schmidt MA, Marcano-Bonilla L, Roberts LR. Gallbladder cancer: Epidemiology and genetic risk associations. Chinese Clinical Oncology. 2019;**8**(4):31

[12] Schnelldorfer T. Porcelain gallbladder: A benign process or concern for malignancy? Journal of Gastrointestinal Surgery. 2013;**17**(6):1161-1168

[13] Lewis JT, Talwalkar JA, Rosen CB, Smyrk TC, Abraham SC. Prevalence and risk factors for gallbladder neoplasia in patients with primary sclerosing cholangitis: Evidence for a metaplasia-dysplasia-carcinoma sequence. The American Journal of Surgical Pathology. 2007;**31**(6):907-913

[14] Dutta U, Poornachandra KS. Gallbladder polyps: How to pick up the sinister ones. Journal of Gastroenterology and Hepatology. 2009;**24**(2):175-178

[15] Razumilava N, Gores GJ, Lindor KD. Cancer surveillance in patients with primary sclerosing cholangitis. Hepatology. 2011;**54**(5):1842-1852

[16] Kumar A, Ali M, Raj V, Kumari A, Rachamalla M, Niyogi S, et al. Arsenic causing gallbladder cancer disease in Bihar. Scientific Reports. 2023;**13**(1):4259

[17] Ganesan N, Bambino K, Boffetta P, Labgaa I. Exploring the potential

carcinogenic role of arsenic in gallbladder cancer. European Journal of Cancer Prevention. 2020;**29**(2):100-109

[18] Chen K, Zhu P, Chen W, Luo K, Shi XJ, Zhai W. Melatonin inhibits proliferation, migration, and invasion by inducing ROS-mediated apoptosis via suppression of the PI3K/Akt/mTOR signaling pathway in gallbladder cancer cells. Aging (Albany NY). 2021;**13**(18):22502

[19] Straif K, Benbrahim-Tallaa L, Baan R, Grosse Y, Secretan B, El Ghissassi F, et al. A review of human carcinogens—Part C: Metals, arsenic, dusts, and fibres. The Lancet Oncology. 2009;**10**(5):453-454

[20] Uesaka K, Yasui K, Morimoto T, Torii A, Yamamura Y, Kodera Y, et al. Visualization of routes of lymphatic drainage of the gallbladder with a carbon particle suspension. Journal of the American College of Surgeons. 1996;**183**(4):345-350

[21] Furlan A, Ferris JV, Hosseinzadeh K, Borhani AA. Gallbladder carcinoma update: Multimodality imaging evaluation, staging, and treatment options. AJR. American Journal of Roentgenology. 2008;**191**:1440-1447

[22] Schwartz LH, Black J, Fong Y, Jarnagin W, Blumgart L, Gruen D, et al. Gallbladder carcinoma: Findings at MR imaging with MR cholangiopancreatography. Journal of Computer Assisted Tomography. 2002;**26**(3):405-410

[23] Gupta P, Dutta U, Rana P, Singhal M, Gulati A, Kalra, et al. Gallbladder reporting and data system (GB-RADS) for risk stratification of gallbladder wall thickening on ultrasonography: An international expert consensus. Abdominal Radiology. 2022;**47**(2):554-565

[24] Siddeek RAT, Gupta A, Gupta S, Goyal B, Gupta AK, Agrawal S, et al. Evaluation of platelet distribution width as novel biomarker in gall bladder cancer. Journal of Carcinogenesis. 2020;**27**(19):5. DOI: 10.4103/jcar.JCar_12_20

[25] Gupta A, Gupta S, Gupta A, Gupta A, Goyal B, Agrawal S, et al. Red cell distribution width: A surrogate biomarker to predict tumor burden in carcinoma gallbladder. Nigerian Journal of Surgery. 2019;**25**(2):198-202

[26] Mani R, Gupta A, Gupta S, Goyal B, Mishra R, Tandon A, et al. Expression of ER, PR, and HER-2 Neu and correlation with tumor markers in gall bladder carcinoma. Journal of Cancer Research and Therapeutics. 2023;**19**(5):1279-1287

[27] Gupta A, Gupta S, Mani R, Durgapal P, Goyal B, Rajput D, et al. Expression of human epidermal growth factor receptor 2, survivin, enhancer of zeste homolog -2, Cyclooxygenase-2, p53 and p16 molecular markers in gall bladder carcinoma. Journal of Carcinogenesis. 2021;**9**(20):7

[28] Sung YN, Song M, Lee JH, et al. Validation of the 8th edition of the American joint committee on cancer staging system for gallbladder cancer and implications for the follow-up of patients without node dissection. Cancer Research and Treatment. 2020;**52**(2):455-468

[29] Dixon E, Vollmer CM Jr, Sahajpal A, et al. An aggressive surgical approach leads to improved survival in patients with gallbladder cancer: A 12-year study at a north American Center. Annals of Surgery. 2005;**241**:385-394

[30] Fuks D, Regimbeau JM, Le Treut YP, et al. Incidental gallbladder cancer by the AFC-GBC-2009 study group. World Journal of Surgery. 2011;**35**:1887-1897

[31] Lee SE, Jang JY, Lim CS, et al. Systematic review on the surgical treatment for T1 gallbladder cancer. World Journal of Gastroenterology. 2011;**17**:174-180

[32] D'Angelica M, Dalal KM, DeMatteo RP, et al. Analysis of the extent of resection for adenocarcinoma of the gallbladder. Annals of Surgical Oncology. 2009;**16**:806-816

[33] Gani F, Buettner S, Margonis GA, et al. Assessing the impact of common bile duct resection in the surgical management of gallbladder cancer. Journal of Surgical Oncology. 2016;**114**:176-180

[34] Pawlik TM, Gleisner AL, Vigano L, et al. Incidence of finding residual disease for incidental gallbladder carcinoma: Implications for re-resection. Journal of Gastrointestinal Surgery. 2007;**11**:1478-1486

[35] Agarwal AK, Kalayarasan R, Javed A, Gupta N, Nag HH. The role of staging laparoscopy in primary gall bladder cancer--an analysis of 409 patients: A prospective study to evaluate the role of staging laparoscopy in the management of gallbladder cancer. Annals of Surgery. 2013;**258**(2):318-323

[36] Tokumitsu Y, Kawaoka T, Matsukuma S, Harada E, Suenaga S, et al. Yamaguchi Pancreatic/Biliary Disease Study Group (YPB). A Prospective Observational Study of Laparoscopic Approaches for Suspected Gallbladder Cancer in Yamaguchi (YPB-002 LAGBY). Updates Surg; 2025

[37] Chee MYM, Wu AGR, Fong KY, Yew A, Koh YX, Goh BKP. Robotic, laparoscopic and open surgery for gallbladder cancer: A systematic review and network meta-analysis. Surgical Endoscopy. 2024;**38**(9):4846-4857

[38] Duffy A, Capanu M, Abou-Alfa GK, Huitzil D, Jarnagin W, Fong Y, et al. Gallbladder cancer (GBC): 10-year experience at memorial Sloan-Kettering cancer centre (MSKCC). Journal of Surgical Oncology. 2008;**98**(7):485-489

[39] Mitin T, Enestvedt CK, Jemal A, Sineshaw HM. Limited use of adjuvant therapy in patients with resected gallbladder cancer despite a strong association with survival. Journal of the National Cancer Institute. 2017;**109**(7):324-326

[40] John NP et al. Capecitabine compared with observation in resected biliary tract cancer (BILCAP): A randomised, controlled, multicentre, phase 3 study primrose. The Lancet Oncology. 2019;**20**(5):663-673

[41] Edeline J, Benabdelghani M, Bertaut A, Watelet J, Hammel P, Joly JP, et al. Gemcitabine and oxaliplatin chemotherapy or surveillance in resected biliary tract cancer (Prodige 12-Accord 18-Unicancer GI): A randomized phase III study. Journal of Clinical Oncology. 2019;**37**(8):658-667. DOI: 10.1200/JCO.18.00050

[42] Valle J, Wasan H, Palmer DH, Cunningham D, Anthoney A, Maraveyas A, et al. ABC-02 trial investigators. Cisplatin plus gemcitabine versus gemcitabine for biliary tract cancer. The New England Journal of Medicine. 2010;**362**(14):1273-1281

[43] Oh DY, He AR, Bouattour M, Okusaka T, Qin S, Chen LT, et al. Durvalumab or placebo plus gemcitabine and cisplatin in participants with advanced biliary tract cancer (TOPAZ-1): Updated overall survival from a randomised phase 3 study. The Lancet Gastroenterology & Hepatology. 2024;**9**(8):694-704

[44] Agrawal S, Singh A, Rahul R, Mishra P, Saxena R. A randomized study of consolidation chemo-radiotherapy versus observation after first-line chemotherapy in advanced gall bladder cancers (RACE-GB study): Trial protocol. International Journal of Clinical Trials. 2023;**10**(1):32-38

Chapter 7

Gallbladder and Bile Ducts: Anatomical Structures and Clinical Associations for 2025

Raimundas Lunevicius

Abstract

This chapter presents a narrative review summarising both classical and contemporary knowledge of gallbladder and bile duct structures, with an emphasis on their clinical associations with cholecystectomy. It provides a comprehensive overview of the biliary anatomy and classification, along with its relevance to surgical safety. Additionally, it focuses on infundibular surgical techniques for laparoscopic cholecystectomy, specifically the subserosal inner (SS-inner) layer and posterior infundibular approaches, which expose the cystic duct and branches or trunk of the cystic artery. Although these techniques appear similar, their anatomical terminology, technical execution, and rationale for avoiding the danger zones vary. Therefore, this chapter explores the theory behind the six-layered gallbladder wall and its relationship with the hepatic plate in a broader context. It emphasises sectional, segmental, and subsegmental (cone unit) Glissonian pedicles, along with the corresponding bile ducts and anchors. Another focus is the classification of bile ducts based on anatomical hierarchy, particularly in relation to the Brisbane 2000 classification and its surgical applications. Enhancing or refreshing the understanding of the intrahepatic and extrahepatic biliary ductal systems is crucial for preventing accidental injuries and reducing morbidity associated with both total and subtotal cholecystectomies.

Keywords: gallbladder, bile duct, anatomy, histology, laparoscopic cholecystectomy, subtotal cholecystectomy, liver surgery, hepatobiliary surgery

1. Introduction

The biliary system (*systema biliaris* in Latin) consists of bile ducts (*ductus biliares*) and the gallbladder (*vesica fellea*). They are large aggregates of tubular structures that vary considerably in terms of volume, length, diameter, anatomical variations, and histological composition. The biliary system originates within the hepatic tissue as an intercellular channel between adjacent hepatocytes, known as *intercellular biliary passages* [1]. This system eventually forms a single bile duct, up to 6 mm in diameter, called the common bile duct (*ductus choledochus*).

Various terms and phrases have been used to describe the biliary system, all of which have clinical and anatomical relevance. For example, the term '*excretory apparatus of the liver'* (*apparatus excretorius hepatis*) emphasises one of the functions of the liver: bile production and its delivery to the duodenum [2]. The stratification of this system into intrahepatic and extrahepatic components follows a logical and anatomical classification. Other commonly used terms include *'biliary tree'* (*arbor biliaris*), *'biliary ductal system'* (*systema ductarius biliaris*), and 'biliary tract' (*tractus biliaris*), which are widely used in both scientific studies and clinical practice [3–9].

Terminology specific to hepatobiliary surgery is often more precise, relying on classifications of liver (*hepar*) anatomy proposed by individual scientists or groups of clinical researchers. For example, the Healey and Schroy segmental and subsegmental nomenclature proposed in 1953 [3] differs from the Couinaud sectorial and segmental nomenclature introduced in 1952 [4]. The Brisbane 2000 system of liver anatomy introduced the term liver section. Consequently, the terminology for some bile ducts was changed again: Couinaud sectorial and Healey-Schroy segmental bile ducts were referred to as sectional bile ducts: anterior (AD) or right anterior (RAD), posterior (PD) or right posterior (RPD), lateral (LD) or left lateral (LLD), and medial (MD) or left medial (LMD).

The Brisbane 2000 classification uniquely emphasises the numerical order division of the liver and, consequently, the bile ducts, which has practical applications in surgical and diagnostic settings [10–12]. Classifying bile ducts based on their anatomical division level is practical and easily understood, especially when the precise name of a bile duct is unclear during preoperative biliary imaging assessment, postoperative debates regarding bile leaks, or unexpected intraoperative events that require precise documentation. This classification system offers the following broad terms: first-order bile duct division (hemiliver level), second-order bile duct division (sectional level), and third-order bile duct division (segmental level).

The gallbladder, as part of the biliary system, is the most stable organ in terms of macroanatomical and microanatomical terminology compared to other biliary structures. However, over the past 15 years, the nomenclature for the cross-sectional anatomy of the gallbladder wall has evolved [13, 14]. It is also important to note that cholecystectomy is one of the most frequently performed abdominal surgical procedures globally. This trend coincides with medicolegal claims related to unexpected or avoidable intra- and postoperative complications [15–19]. Consequently, maintaining accuracy in every phase of surgical care, including documentation, is essential.

Surgeons performing cholecystectomies often use jargon when discussing the gross anatomy of the gallbladder and its cross-sectional wall structure.

However, emerging theories regarding the composition of the peritoneal and hepatic walls of the gallbladder, as well as the detailed anatomical relationship between the gallbladder wall layers and the hepatic hilar system, are essential for promoting a culture of safety in cholecystectomy and ensuring the correct use of anatomical terminology. Furthermore, translating certain terms from the Brisbane 2000 consensus meeting, such as section, sector, and segment, into other languages [20], including medical Latin, presents challenges because of their linguistic similarities impacting international surgical communication.

This chapter summarises both historical and contemporary knowledge regarding the anatomical structure of the gallbladder and bile ducts, with a particular focus on their relevance to cholecystectomy-related clinical practices. The main objective of this study is to establish an educational resource for medical students, residents, fellows, researchers, nurses, licenced surgeons, physicians, and diagnosticians. This resource aims to reinforce the idea that cholecystectomy extends beyond the operating theatre, encompassing how surgeons discuss, document, report, teach, and share their experiences.

2. Methods

A predefined chapter plan was developed following an agreement to contribute to this project. Literature sources for each section and subsection of the chapter were carefully selected using the PubMed bibliographic database (https://pubmed.ncbi.nlm.nih.gov), Google (https://www.google.co.uk/client=safari), and Google Scholar (https://scholar.google.com). In addition to these online resources, relevant literature was obtained from hospital and private libraries and from research and audit projects conducted by the author. This chapter follows six key elements of narrative review articles [21], with basic anatomical terms provided in Latin in parentheses. The third section, which focuses on eponyms, is primarily based on secondary literature sources, except for one study [4].

To classify atypical anatomical variants and surgical complications, five categories were established according to their frequency of occurrence. Conditions classified as 'very common' have a risk of ≥10%, affecting >1 in 10 individuals. 'Common' conditions have a risk between 1 and 10%, affecting between 1 in 10 and 1 in 100 individuals. 'Uncommon' conditions have a risk ranging from 0.1 to 1%, affecting between 1 in 100 and 1 in 1000 individuals. 'Rare' conditions fall within a risk range of 0.01 to 0.1%, affecting between 1 in 1000 and 1 in 10,000 individuals. Finally, 'very rare' conditions have a risk of <0.01%, often appearing only as isolated reports where the absolute risk is unknown or cannot be quantified, affecting <1 in 10,000 individuals [22].

Although clinical scenarios were used sparingly, they were included to support specific statements. This chapter also presents original figures and tables. It is part of the open-access book project 'Hepatobiliary Medicine and Surgery—Gallbladder' (ISBN 978-1-83,635-270-9) published by IntechOpen (https://www.intechopen.com).

3. Eponyms

Eponyms in hepatobiliary surgery can be categorised chronologically [23], by organ or anatomical subsystem (liver, gallbladder, and bile ducts), or by anatomical classification (systematic anatomy vs. operative anatomy and microanatomy vs. macroanatomy) [8, 24]. Subsections 3.1–3.13 detail eponymous terms relevant to biliary surgery, some of which are also associated with hepatic surgery.

3.1 Glissonian (Walean) pedicle

In 1640, Johannes Walaeus (1604–1649) was the first to describe the common vascular biliary sheath, which includes three key structures: the portal vein, hepatic artery, and the bile duct. In 1654, Francis Glisson (1597–1677) provided a comprehensive description of this sheath [9]. Consequently, the connective tissue layer surrounding the portal triad is known as the Glissonian sheath.

The Glissonian pedicle consists of a portal triad and its sheath and is classified into extrahepatic and intrahepatic types.

3.2 Laënnec's capsule

In 1802, René Théophile Hyacinthe Laënnec (1781–1826), the physician who invented the stethoscope and coined the term micronodular cirrhosis, first described a distinct membrane surrounding the entire liver parenchyma, including the areas where the gallbladder and diaphragm attach. This dense fibrous layer beneath the liver's serosa is known as Laënnec's capsule. This is not equivalent to the liver serosa, which is an independent structural layer partially covering Laënnec's capsule.

During laparoscopic cholecystectomy, a thin, shiny, fibrous layer may be visible in the gallbladder bed. This layer represents Laënnec's capsule, which separates the cystic plate of the gallbladder from the liver parenchyma. If exposed during surgery, it indicates damage to the cystic plate, suggesting that the dissection plane was too deep.

Laënnec's capsule extends into the liver hilum, forming the outer layer of the intrahepatic Glissonian (Walean) pedicles. On the opposite side of the liver, it forms the outer layer of the major hepatic veins and their tributaries [25, 26].

3.3 Couinaud's hepatic plates

Claude Couinaud (1922–2008) established the concept of the liver plate system, a fibrous layer that covers Laënnec's capsule at key anatomical sites on the inferior surface of the liver. It is considered a single anatomical entity, along with the sectional and liversegment 1 Glissonian sheaths [4, 25].

3.4 Hartmann's pouch

Hartmann's pouch, described by Henri Albert Hartmann (1860–1952) but first noted by Broca, is situated between the peritoneal wall of the body and the neck of the gallbladder. It is typically observed in diseased gallbladders [27]. It is important to mention that this pouch is absent in healthy, normal-volume gallbladders [2].

Excessive traction on Hartmann's pouch is one of the most common causes of portal vein injury, which can lead to catastrophic bleeding. It can also cause necrosis-related disruption of the cystic duct (CD).

3.5 Lütkens' sphincter

First described in 1926 by Ulrich Lütkens, this sphincter was originally thought to be a circular bundle of smooth muscle fibres located at the junction of the gallbladder neck (Gn) and CD. Other anatomists from the seventeenth and nineteenth centuries, including Glisson and Heister, have also documented its existence. However, the current literature suggests that a consistent anatomical sphincter in the gallbladder outflow tract is unlikely to exist [28, 29].

3.6 Heister's valves

Owing to their morphological appearance and function within the CD, cystic valves are also known as the spiral valves of Heister. These structures were named after Lorenz Heister (1683–1758), who first described them in 1732. Notably, the morphology of the cystic valves does not follow a consistent pattern [30].

3.7 Rokitansky-Aschoff sinuses

Rokitansky-Aschoff sinuses are outpouchings of the gallbladder mucosa into the fibromuscular layer, a condition also referred to as intramural diverticulosis [2, 6]. These sinuses were named after the pathologists who identified them: Karl Freiherr von Rokitansky (1804–1878) and Karl Albert Ludwig Aschoff (1866–1942).

In patients with acute severe cholecystitis classified as Tokyo grade 2 or 3 [31–33], infectious pathogens may invade the mucosal sinuses, leading to localised perforation, pus accumulation, or infected necrotic tissue within the subserosal layer of the hepatic wall of the gallbladder. If the abscess extends beyond the cystic plate and Laënnec's capsule, it may potentially spread into the adjacent liver parenchyma.

3.8 Rouvière sulcus

The Rouvière sulcus, named after Henri Rouvière (1876–1952), was first described in 1924. It varies in length (2–5 cm), width (a few millimetres to 2 cm), and depth. This sulcus appears as a horizontal groove on the inferior surface of the liver [34, 35]. However, the sulcus may be absent in 10% of patients.

The Rouvière sulcus is bordered by two edges: superior (ventral) and inferior (dorsal). It is a surgical landmark between the right hemiliver (S5) and caudate process (segment 1 of the liver). Therefore, the Rouvière sulcus is also known as the sulcus of the caudate process. In many patients, a tubular structure at the bottom of the sulcus represents a subsegmental S6A Glissonian pedicle [36].

The area between the distal Rouvière sulcus and the lower serosa of the gallbladder is considered a no-touch zone because of the risk of injuring the components of the right posterior Glissonian pedicle (Gpost) and possibly G1C (Glissonian pedicle for the caudate process of liver segment 1) during cholecystectomy. Similarly, the right anterior Glissonian pedicle lies on the opposite side of the gallbladder (left side) at its lowest point, where the cystic plate merges with the hilar plate in segment 4. This area is also considered a no-touch zone.

The Rouvière sulcus is a key lateral reference point for safe gallbladder surgery [34]. When the gallbladder is elevated toward the diaphragm, the inferior border of safe dissection should be positioned above an imaginary diagonal line (R4U) extending between the medial angle of the Rouvière sulcus and the lower edge of liver segment 4. However, gallbladder surgery should not rely solely on imaging.

3.9 Calot's triangle

Calot's triangle, named after Jean-François Calot (1861–1944), was first described in 1891. It is geometrically bordered by the cystic artery, CD, and common hepatic duct. The cystic lymph node, also known as Lund's or Mascagni's node, is a sentinel lymph node of the gallbladder, typically located anterior to or within the plane of Calot's triangle [37].

3.10 Rex-Cantlie line

In 1888, Rex (1861–1936) introduced the concept of two hemilivers based on the anatomy of the portal vein and its branches. A decade later, in 1897, James Cantlie (1851–1926) published his observations on a line that divides the liver into right and left halves [38, 39].

The imaginary Rex-Cantlie line extends from the centre of the gallbladder bed to the inferior vena cava, forming an almost flat plane for right and left hepatectomies [4]. The middle hepatic vein or its significant tributaries within liver segments 4 and 5 may be closely related to the intrahepatic gallbladder in some anatomical cases. In such situations, the safest approach, subtotal cholecystectomy (STC), must be considered. The Rex-Cantlie-Serege line is another eponymous version of this reference line [30].

3.11 Luschka duct

Luschka ducts are identified in 5–6% of patients (1 in 20 cases). They do not cross the segmental border of the liver (S5B). These ducts may traverse the gallbladder fossa and fuse with either the right or common hepatic duct, as described by Hubert von Luschka (1820–1875) in 1863. The upstream end of the duct of Luschka is typically found on the cystic plate; however, it is not connected to the gallbladder.

Although injury to the Luschka duct can be generally avoided during conventional cholecystectomy, there remains a risk of damage when the duct merges with the common hepatic duct, particularly during right hepatectomy or cholecystectomy [40]. Some practical implications are associated with gallbladder surgical techniques. For instance, the continuous use of diathermy on the posterior subserosa, or inadvertently on the cystic plate or deeper tissues without adequate blunt dissection, exposure, or identification of the bundles of the SS-outer layer, may result in injury to the Luschka duct.

Alternative terms for the duct of Luschka include the subvesical duct (commonly referenced in the scientific literature) and supravesical duct. The term accessory (or aberrant) bile ducts is also used to describe Luschka ducts.

3.12 Winsløw's foramen

The epiploic foramen (*foramen epiploicum*) is an anatomical passage that connects the lesser and greater sacs of the peritoneal cavity. It is named after Jacob Benignus Winsløw (1669–1760) [41]. Among the various surgical implications related to foramen anatomy, two are particularly significant. First, the tip of the subhepatic drain should be positioned anterior to Winsløw's foramen. Second, Winsløw's foramen plays a critical role in the precise placement of a vascular clamp on the hepatoduodenal ligament to control bleeding from the portal vein, its branches, or liver parenchyma (the Pringle manoeuvre).

3.13 Other eponymous terms

Several eponymous terms are frequently used in biliary surgery, particularly when discussing postoperative complications such as fluid accumulation in the peritoneal cavity and obstructive jaundice. These include Morrison's pouch (the hepatorenal recess, named after Rutherford Morrison [1853–1939]), the ampulla of Vater (the great duodenal papilla, named after Abraham Vater [1684–1751]), the Oddi sphincter (first described in 1887 by Ruggero Oddi [1864–1913]), and the Wirsung duct, named after Johann Georg Wirsung (1589–1643) in 1642, which connects to the common bile duct in only two-thirds of individuals.

4. Conventional description of gallbladder morphology

The structure of the gallbladder is similar in humans and other mammals [29]. Its size and wall thickness depend on the physiological cycle of bile storage and emptying.

4.1 Gross anatomy

The gallbladder is a hollow, mesoperitoneal organ with a piriform shape situated in a relatively flat fossa on the inferior surface of the liver. It is connected to the biliary tract *via* a single CD. In adults, the gallbladder typically measures 7.5–10 cm in length and 3–4 cm in width, with a capacity of 40–50 ml of bile.

The gallbladder is arbitrarily divided into three portions: the fundus (*fundus vesicae felleae*), body (*corpus vesicae felleae*), and neck (*collum vesicae felleae*). No fixed anatomical lines or planes define their borders. The visceral peritoneum covers the fundus (part of the gallbladder that extends beyond the anterior margin of the liver) when the anatomy of the gallbladder is standard. In the surgical literature, the fundus is also referred to as 'domus' (e.g., '*domus-down cholecystectomy technique*'). In contrast, the visceral peritoneum only partially covered the gallbladder body (Gb) and Gn. The Gn begins where the organ narrows and measures 5–7 mm in length. At the orifice of the CD, the mucosal folds of the gallbladder converge to form oblique ridges that extend into the CD as the spiral valves of Heister.

The part of the gallbladder wall that is not covered by the visceral peritoneum is called the hepatic wall (*paries hepaticus vesicae felleae*). The remaining part is termed the peritoneal wall (*paries peritonealis vesicae felleae*). The standard hepatic-to-peritoneal wall ratio is 30:70. In gallbladder surgery, the terms '*anterior wall*' and '*posterior wall*' are widely used as surgical jargon, although they are practical for surgical planning. **Figure 1** shows transabdominal ultrasonograms of a normal gallbladder (**Figure 1A**) and a gallbladder containing an asymptomatic incidental gallstone (**Figure 1B**).

Understanding the standard ratio between the two walls of the gallbladder is essential for estimating the percentage of gallbladder excised during STC. This procedure is often performed under challenging conditions to minimise the risk of injury to the ductal, vascular, intestinal, gastric, and diaphragmatic structures associated with conventional cholecystectomy. In the surgical literature, STC is commonly referred to as 'partial cholecystectomy', as this term is used in the classifications of surgical

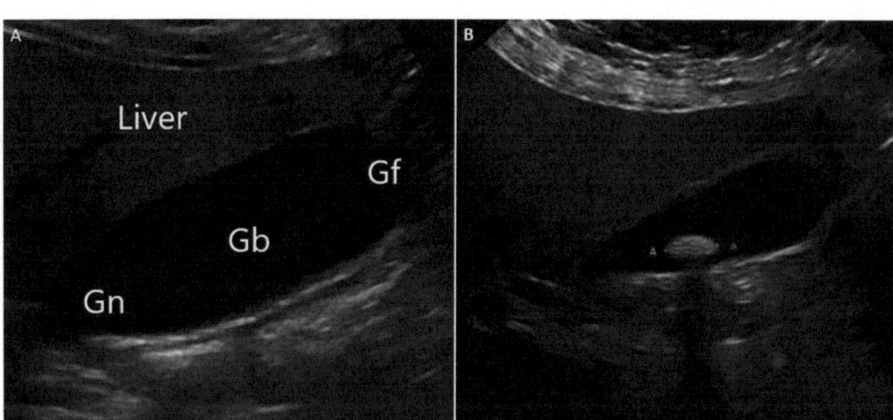

Figure 1.
Transabdominal ultrasonograms of the gallbladder. A: The gallbladder is a sonolucent, thin-walled hollow organ devoid of acoustic shadows. B: An incidental gallstone detected in a symptom-free patient, showing an acoustic shadow beneath the calculus. Abbreviations: Gf = gallbladder fundus; Gb = gallbladder body; Gn = gallbladder neck.

procedures and interventions, such as the Office of Population Censuses and Surveys Classification of Interventions and Procedures, Version 4, and *Current Procedural Terminology®* [42, 43].

Hartmann's pouch is the most common site of gallstone impaction within the gallbladder cavity. As it overlaps with the CD, it serves as a key surgical landmark for identifying the CD in both open and laparoscopic surgeries.

The close anatomical relationship between the gallbladder fundus (Gf) and anterior abdominal wall explains most clinical symptoms and signs associated with cholecystitis or pathological gallbladder distention. The fundus extends 1 cm beyond the anterior margin of the liver and is positioned at the apex of the angle formed by the ninth rib and the lateral border of the right rectus muscle. It contacts the parietal peritoneum of the anterior abdominal wall. When markedly distended, the gallbladder becomes palpable [5]. This phenomenon is referred to as Courvoisier's sign, which was first described by Ludwig Georg Courvoisier in 1890. However, the position and topography of the gallbladder can vary depending on factors such as liver size, degree of gallbladder distention, and any acquired or congenital conditions affecting the diaphragm. **Figure 2** illustrates an atypical gallbladder location in a patient with no documented history of trauma or right-sided diaphragmatic disease (sporadic case).

4.2 Wall structure

The wall of a healthy gallbladder typically measures 1–2 mm in thickness, although this can vary depending on the degree of physiological gallbladder distention. It consists of three distinct layers: the mucosa, muscular layer (often referred to as the fibromuscular layer), and either serosa, which includes subserosal connective tissue for the peritoneal wall, or adventitia, composed of alveolar connective tissue for the hepatic wall of the gallbladder. Notably, the definition of gallbladder adventitia varies.

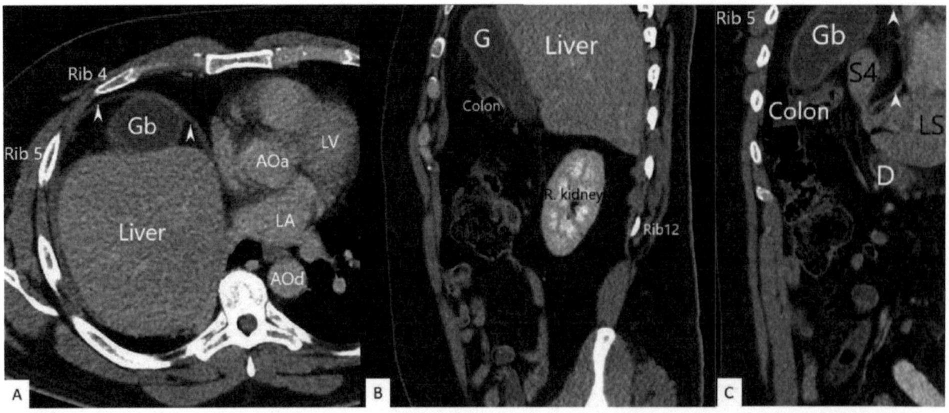

Figure 2.
The gallbladder body and right diaphragm are located anteriorly at the level of the fourth right rib, aligning with a zone along the mid-clavicular line. The thick-walled gallbladder is positioned well above the right kidney at the horizontal level of the base of the heart. The transverse colon encircles the neck and part of the gallbladder body. The patient was admitted as an emergency case with acute calculous cholecystitis. Computed tomography images include selected views: axial (A), sagittal (B), and coronal (C). The diaphragm appears intact, with no signs of liver protrusion into the chest cavity. Abbreviations: A: Gb = gallbladder body; AOa = ascending aorta; AOd = descending aorta; LV = left ventricle; LA = left atrium (with the left pulmonary vein). B: G = gallbladder. C: Gb = gallbladder body; S4 = liver segment 4; LS = lateral section, left hemiliver; D = duodenum. Four arrowheads (two in A and two in C) indicate the right-sided diaphragm.

For instance, a cystic plate can be regarded as part of the adventitia because it is a layer of connective tissue.

4.2.1 Outer layer: Serosa or adventitia

The outer layer of the peritoneal wall of the gallbladder is the serosa (*tunica serosa vesicae felleae*), which is formed by the visceral peritoneum. Beneath the mesothelium and basement membrane, the subserosal layer consists of fatty tissue (loose connective tissue), arteries, veins, lymphatics, nerves, and paraganglia, along with fibrous and elastic tissue that forms the matrix for this layer.

The adventitia (*tunica adventitia vesicae felleae*) is the outermost layer of the hepatic wall of the gallbladder and consists of areolar connective tissue that connects the gallbladder to the cystic plate. This layer is particularly rich in fibrous connective tissue.

Conventionally, during cholecystectomy, the hepatic wall of the gallbladder should be dissected through the areolar connective tissue, as it serves as the appropriate surgical plane for the procedure. Deviating from this guideline (too close to the gallbladder or liver) is considered improper.

4.2.2 Middle layer: Muscular (fibromuscular or muscularis propria)

The muscular layer (*tunica muscularis vesicae felleae*) of the gallbladder exhibits a distinct morphological composition of smooth muscle fibres. Myocyte bundles within this layer are loosely arranged in three orientations: longitudinal, circular, and oblique. As there is no strict pattern in this layer, unlike the gastrointestinal tract (two layers), it resembles the muscularis propria of the mucosa. In addition, Cajal-like cells have been identified within the fibro-muscular layer of the gallbladder [44]. Although the precise function of these cells remains unclear, they are similar to the interstitial cells of Cajal, which act as pacemakers in the muscular layer of the digestive tract.

4.2.3 Inner layer: Mucosa

The mucosa (*tunica mucosa vesicae felleae*) of the gallbladder has a distinct honeycomb-like appearance. It is composed of a single layer of columnar epithelial cells with microvilli supported by a basement membrane and subepithelial layer. Columnar epithelial cells, which measure 15–25 μm in height, are covered with microvilli that range from 0.2 to 0.5 μm in length. These cells are coated with a glycocalyx layer, which contains mucus granules that protect the epithelial cells from bile salts. In addition, basal cells measuring 10–15 μm in diameter have been identified between the epithelial cells of the mucosa [29].

The subepithelial layer, which is loosely attached to the muscular layer, contains numerous elastic fibres, lymphatic vessels, extensive microvasculature, and a ganglionated plexus. Consequently, separating the necrotic mucosa from the fibromuscular layer of the hepatic wall during STC is a relatively straightforward surgical step.

Only the Gn contains tubular alveolar glands within the subepithelial layer. In addition, unlike the gastrointestinal tract, the gallbladder mucosa lacks a muscularis propria, which means that it does not have a submucosal layer. A distinct characteristic of gallbladder walls is the presence of Rokitansky-Aschoff sinuses, which are involved in the extraluminal spread of gallbladder infections and may serve as potential sites for cholecystomicrolithiasis.

5. Gallbladder anatomy and structure: An update

5.1 The fundamentals

The fundamentals of gross anatomy remain unchanged. However, two key features should be highlighted. First, the line connecting the centre of the fundus to the CD on the gallbladder peritoneal wall divides it into two equal parts: anterior and posterior. This division enables surgeons and pathologists to accurately describe the anatomical locations of unexpected (perforation) and expected (tumour) findings. This is particularly relevant for oncological surgeries [45, 46]. Second, modern biliary anatomy is characterised by the precise topographical relationship between the gallbladder wall, bile ducts (in order of division), and anchors. The term '*peritoneal wall of the gallbladder*' is synonymous with '*visceral wall of the gallbladder*'; however, the former is the preferred term.

5.2 Surgical cross-sectional structure

The peritoneal and hepatic walls of the gallbladder consist of an unequal number of layers: five and six, respectively [13, 47–50].

5.2.1 Five layers of the peritoneal wall

The layers of the peritoneal wall, from the inside to the outside, are as follows: mucosa (first layer), fibromuscular layer (second layer), inner subserosa (third layer, abbreviated as SS-inner), outer subserosa (fourth layer, abbreviated as SS-outer), and serosa (fifth layer). A distinctive feature of this cross-sectional anatomical system is the division of the subserosal layer into two distinct histological layers: the SS-inner and SS-outer. The serosa consists solely of mesothelium and basement membrane. The SS-outer layer contains abundant fatty tissue and sparse blood vessels, resembling areolar tissue. In contrast, the SS-inner layer is rich in vasculature and fibrous tissue and is firmly attached to the fibromuscular layer of the gallbladder [13, 14, 51].

5.2.1.1 Practical implications related to the peritoneal wall

During conventional cholecystectomy, the SS-outer (fourth) layer should be exposed after incising the serosa of the peritoneal wall of the gallbladder at the lower body level, or if the anatomy is clear, on the surface of the Gn. Further division of the gallbladder peritoneal wall between the SS-outer (fourth) and SS-inner (third) layers is considered safe.

However, owing to the close histological and physiological relationships between the SS-inner and the fibromuscular (second) layer, safely separating these layers is not feasible. Attempting to do so can lead to iatrogenic perforation of the gallbladder or CD.

To prevent accidental thermal injury to the bile ducts and gallbladder, the use of high-frequency alternate-polarity electric currents should be minimised or completely avoided during tissue coagulation and division (using laparoscopic scissors and a dissector).

A Glissonian pedicle is often observed at the base of the Rouvière sulcus (**Figure 3**). As mentioned in Section 3.8 (Eponyms), it represents a fourth-order

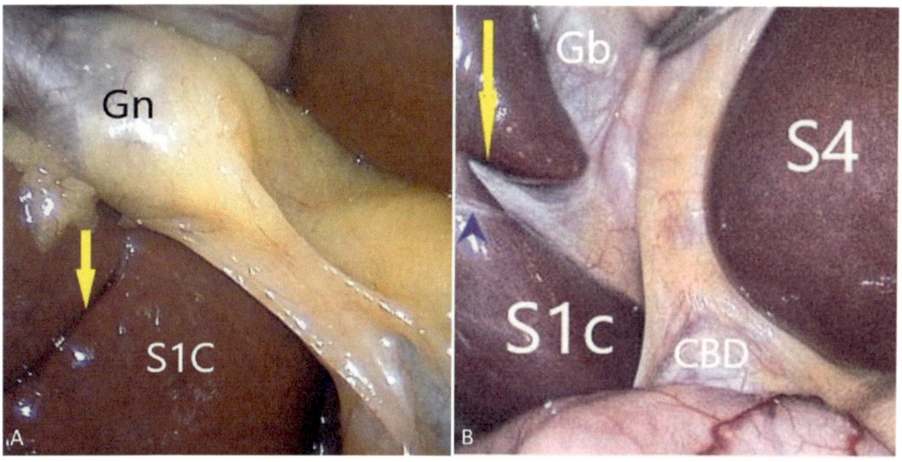

Figure 3.
Rouvière sulcus (see arrows). A: Standard size and appearance. B: Glissonian pedicle at the bottom of the sulcus, usually G6A (B6A). The blue arrowhead points to the tubular structure, the anchor. Abbreviations: Gn = neck of the gallbladder; S1C = caudate process of liver segment 1; Gb = body of the gallbladder; S4 = liver segment 4; CBD = common bile duct.

division Glissonian pedicle (G6A) with a bile duct B6A within it [36]. Extra caution is necessary when performing a posterior serosal incision and during separation of the SS-outer and SS-inner layers.

5.2.2 Hepatic wall

The hepatic wall consists of six layers, from inside to outside: the mucosa (first layer), fibromuscular layer (second layer), SS-inner layer (third layer), SS-outer layer (fourth layer), cystic plate (fifth layer), and Laënnec's capsule, also known as Laënnec's membrane (sixth layer). The mucosa, fibromuscular, SS-inner, and SS-outer layers are identical to the corresponding layers in the peritoneal wall of the gallbladder. However, the SS-outer layer (fourth layer of the hepatic wall) and cystic plate (fifth layer) are thicker proximally and thinner distally. The cystic plate extends from the sectional Glissonian (Walean) sheaths to Laënnec's capsule within the bed area of the gallbladder. A narrow gap exists between the cystic plate and the Laënnec's capsule [13, 51].

5.2.2.1 Gallbladder's bed and cystic fossa

The term '*gallbladder's bed*' refers to the fibrous connective tissue that attaches the gallbladder to the liver. This is conventionally known as cystic plate. Conversely, the cystic fossa is a small area on the inferior surface of the liver (covered by Laënnec's capsule) between the right and left hemilivers, where the gallbladder is situated. This part of the inferior surface resembles a shallow depression, as described by the anatomists [1, 2, 7]. However, sometimes it may be deep [7].

5.2.2.2 Practical implications related to the anatomy of the hepatic wall

The anatomy and topography of the first- and second-order divisions of the extrahepatic bile ducts and their variants must be carefully considered when ablating tissues within and from the hepatocystic region. In conventional 3-layer cholecystectomy, the space between the outer and inner SS layers is referred to as the '*Right plane*'.

The cystic plate, a fibrous layer beneath the outer SS layer, is easily recognisable. In contrast, Laënnec's capsule is very thin and difficult to identify, even during laparoscopic cholecystectomy in patients with typical hepatobiliary anatomy. Laënnec's capsule appears as a small, glistening layer of fibrous tissue. When a surgeon observes a shiny liver surface during cholecystectomy, it is crucial to pause, as this indicates Laënnec's capsule, the gateway to the liver parenchyma or intrahepatic anatomical structures. This serves as a warning of potential surgical risks.

The most common extrahepatic bile duct relevant for cholecystectomy is the right infraportal PD [52–54]. This duct runs close to the medial aspect of the Rouvière sulcus (when present). Ideally, the course of the GDA should be identified before surgery using bile duct imaging techniques, such as contrast-enhanced computed tomography cholangiography, magnetic resonance cholangiography, or, when indicated, endoscopic retrograde cholangiopancreatography.

When performing a conventional cholecystectomy on a patient with a confirmed diagnosis of benign symptomatic or complicated gallstone disease based solely on an ultrasound scan, PD variation should always be considered. The duct is at risk of damage when the proximal portion of the gallbladder is separated from severely inflamed tissues in the hepatocystic region.

A partially intrahepatic gallbladder is another risk factor. Given its topographical relationship with the RAD, the same principle of surgical safety should be applied when operating on the anterior (medial) side of the proximal gallbladder and cystic pedicle.

6. Function

Bile is a physiological fluid produced by the liver at a rate of approximately 1 L every 24 h that aids in the digestion of dietary fats. Bile acids constitute two-thirds of the bile.

The primary function of the gallbladder is to store, concentrate, and release bile between meals *via* contractions of the common bile duct and duodenum. Spiral valves in the CD are essential for bile accumulation, retention, and storage. Within 2–3 h, the gallbladder concentrates the stored bile to as little as one-tenth of its original volume. However, when the stored bile volume exceeds 100 mL, the fibromuscular layer of the gallbladder contracts, the sphincter of Oddi relaxes, and bile is released into the duodenum through the common bile duct and hepatopancreatic ampulla, which lack peristaltic activity.

6.1 Regulation

6.1.1 Motility

Broadly speaking, extrinsic and intrinsic innervation, along with humoral factors and neuropeptides, modulate the motility of the gallbladder and, consequently, its primary function [55, 56]. Extrinsic innervation includes the right phrenic nerve, right vagus nerve (through its hepatic branch), and celiac plexus, which are associated with spinal nerves T7–9. The intrinsic innervation system consists of ganglionated plexuses within the gallbladder wall.

DOI: http://dx.doi.org/10.5772/intechopen.1011304

More specifically, the motor function of the gallbladder is regulated by bile acids acting through the bile duct receptor TGR5, as well as by neurohumoral molecules such as cholecystokinin and fibroblast growth factor (FGF15/19), which are released from endocrine cells of the duodenal mucosa into the bloodstream. These signals trigger gallbladder contraction and emptying in response to dietary fat in the duodenal lumen [29]. Notably, TGR5 refers to Takeda G protein-coupled receptor 5 [57], whereas FGF15 (in mice) and FGF19 (in humans) play a role in bile acid metabolism [58].

6.1.2 Concentration

The physiological mechanisms underlying bile accumulation are unique and are driven by the dynamic balance between the absorptive and secretory functions of the gallbladder mucosa, which fluctuates with feeding cycles. The key to bile concentration lies in the passive movement of water and active absorption of electrolytes from bile into intercellular spaces, which are then transported to capillaries in the subepithelial layer.

Epithelial cells of the gallbladder mucosa secrete glycocalyx (a mucinous coating that protects the cell surface) and bicarbonate, which is a physiological cytoprotective biochemical substance that shields the gallbladder mucosa from bile acids. Glycocalyx secretion is stimulated by calcium-dependent pathways activated by adenosine triphosphate (ATP). In addition, vasoactive intestinal peptides released after feeding stimulate bicarbonate secretion by gallbladder epithelial cells *via* a cyclic adenosine monophosphate (cAMP)-dependent pathway [29].

6.2 Associations with clinical practice

Changes in the motor function of the gallbladder can impair its protective functions and alter the chemical composition of bile acids, contributing to gallstone disease. Conversely, cholecystectomy may lead to nonspecific and specific gastrointestinal symptoms, especially in patients with pre-existing functional gastrointestinal syndromes, such as duodenogastric reflux or irritable bowel syndrome, or following resection of the distal small intestine (where 95% of bile salts are reabsorbed) and the colon. Furthermore, cholecystectomy increases enterohepatic recirculation rates of bile acids, which can result in adverse metabolic effects and an increased risk of fatty liver disease, cirrhosis, and small bowel carcinoids, independent of gallstone disease.

Gallbladder dysmotility is typically defined as a gallbladder ejection fraction of less than 35% on scintigraphy [59]. However, the clinical significance of this criterion must be carefully assessed in the context of surgery for functional gallbladder disorders. It is essential to evaluate symptoms using the Rome IV criteria and rule out functional biliary obstruction due to sphincter of Oddi dysfunction or idiopathic recurrent pancreatitis [60]. Multidisciplinary shared decision-making is crucial.

7. Congenital anomalies of the gallbladder

Developmental anomalies of the gallbladder can be classified into two categories: locational and structural. Although locational deviations from the norm are uncommon or rare, structural anomalies are exceedingly rare, with the exception of a condition known as the *'Phrygian cap'* [5, 61]. **Table 1** summarises the 12 congenital gallbladder anomalies.

Item	Congenital anomalies	Definition and incidence
	Locational	
1	Intrahepatic	
	Partially	A common condition when a peritoneal wall to hepatic wall ratio is less than 7 to 3.
	Completely	Entirely intrahepatic gallbladder; rare or very rare.
2	Sinistroposition	A type of malposition. On the left side from the falciform ligament, as shown in **Figure 4**. An estimated incidence rate of the left-sided gallbladder is <0.3% [62].
3	Medioposition	A type of malposition. On the right side from the falciform ligament but displaced medially to the base on liver segment 4, as shown in **Figure 5** [63].
	Structural	
4	The folded fundus	It is the most common congenital gallbladder anomaly, with an incidence of 4% (range, 1–6%). This anomaly is known as a '*Phrygian cap*'. Some texts describe it as an acquired condition with an abundance of fibrotic tissue [5, 61].
5	Ectopic liver tissue on or within the gallbladder	The estimated incidence is approximately ≤0.3% [64].
6	A double gallbladder:	Sporadic anomaly.
	with conjoined cystic duct	—
	with two cystic ducts	—
7	Bilobed gallbladder:	Sporadic anomaly.
	longitudinal	The septum within the gallbladder cavity is longitudinal.
	transverse	The septum is transverse.
8	Multiseptated gallbladder	MSG, 'honeycomb gallbladder' [65].
9	Absence of the gallbladder:	Sporadic anomaly; incorporates three conditions. Incidence, 0.035–0.3% [29].
	agenesis	—
	aplasia	—
	hypoplasia	—
10	Agenesis of the cystic duct	Sporadic anomaly. The direct fusion of the gallbladder and common hepatic duct.
11	Diverticulum	Sporadic anomaly. It involves all layers of the gallbladder.
12	Ectopic pancreas tissue	Rare. A cause of nonspecific symptoms. Malignant transformation possible [66].

Table 1.
Principal congenital anomalies of the gallbladder.

The practical implications associated with developmental anomalies of the gallbladder should be considered before and during cholecystectomy.

The terms 'intrahepatic gallbladder' and 'pseudointrahepatic gallbladder' denote two distinct concepts. A pseudointrahepatic gallbladder is an acquired condition observed in patients with hepatomegaly owing to various factors. In such instances,

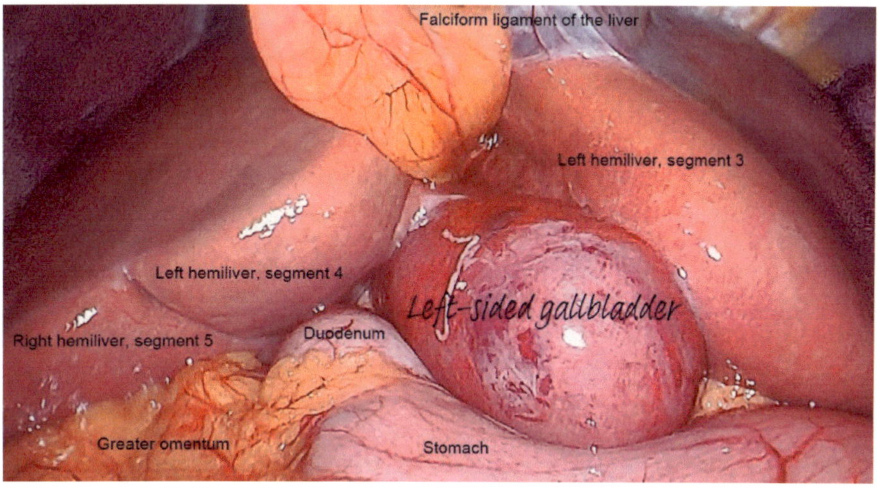

Figure 4.
Laparoscopic inspection: a left-sided gallbladder, acute cholecystitis. The fissure on the visceral surface of the liver (right side) can be interpreted as an external hallmark of the Rex-Cantlie-Serege plane, separating the right hemiliver from the left hemiliver. This figure is part of the open-access article [62], distributed under the Creative Commons Attribution Licence (CC BY-NC 4.0). This licence permits unrestricted use, distribution, and reproduction of the article's material in any medium, provided that the original work is properly cited.

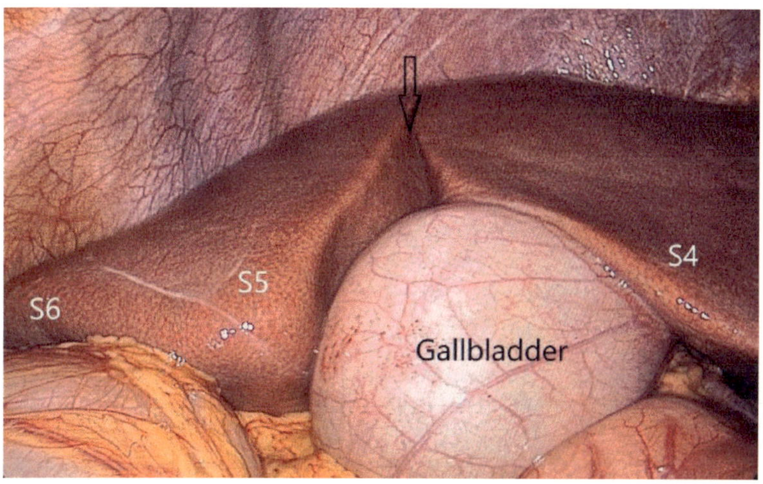

Figure 5.
Medioposition, gallbladder. It is attached to segment 4 of the left hemiliver. A large groove (fissure) is visible on the superior surface of the liver (arrow), positioned to the right of the gallbladder. The direction of this fissure does not correspond with the Rex-Cantlie line. Abbreviations: S4 = liver segment 4; S5 = liver segment 5; S6 = liver segment 6.

the ratio of the peritoneal wall to the hepatic wall remains 7:3. However, the difficulty of cholecystectomy is often at the maximum degree or score owing to the depth of the gallbladder bed and, hence, the gallbladder.

Second, congenital gallbladder malformations are often associated with anatomical variations in the biliary ductal and portal systems. This is especially relevant when performing surgeries on patients with left-sided gallbladders [62].

Third, although a 'Phrygian cap' as a gallbladder's structural condition has no clinical significance, certain diagnostic differentials, such as fundal adenomyomatosis or adenoma of the fundus, should be considered. Fourth, if the ectopic liver tissue is connected to the gallbladder, the junction between these tissues should be clipped, Hem-o-loked, or ligated to prevent bile leakage, when possible. Fifth, patients with gallbladder agenesis may present with symptoms of gallstone disease affecting CDs.

Sixth, congenital malformations of the gallbladder and CD are associated with a high surgical risk [67]. All surgical options, including abandoning cholecystectomy [68] and STC [62], should be considered to prevent iatrogenic injuries during surgery. This consideration is particularly pertinent in emergency and urgent general surgery contexts [62].

8. Cystic pedicle

The cystic pedicle is a fold of pericholecystic tissue located between the medial aspect of the cystic plate superiorly and the visceral peritoneum covering the CD, inferiorly. It is bordered by the common hepatic duct medially, the hepatic wall of the Gn laterally, and the visceral peritoneum both anteriorly and posteriorly (**Figure 6**). Within this fold, the adipose tissue (similar in appearance to the SS-outer layer of the gallbladder) serves as a medium containing the cystic artery (or arteries), CDs, veins, and lymph nodes.

Calot's triangle is part of the cystic pedicle and hepatocystic area. The hepatocystic area extends laterally beyond the cystic artery, forming a larger anatomical space than Calot's triangle. Although it lacks a lateral landmark, the angle formed between the proximal third of the hepatic wall and the cystic plate roughly defines the hepatocystic area, often referred to as the hepatocystic triangle, to simplify the surgical terminology.

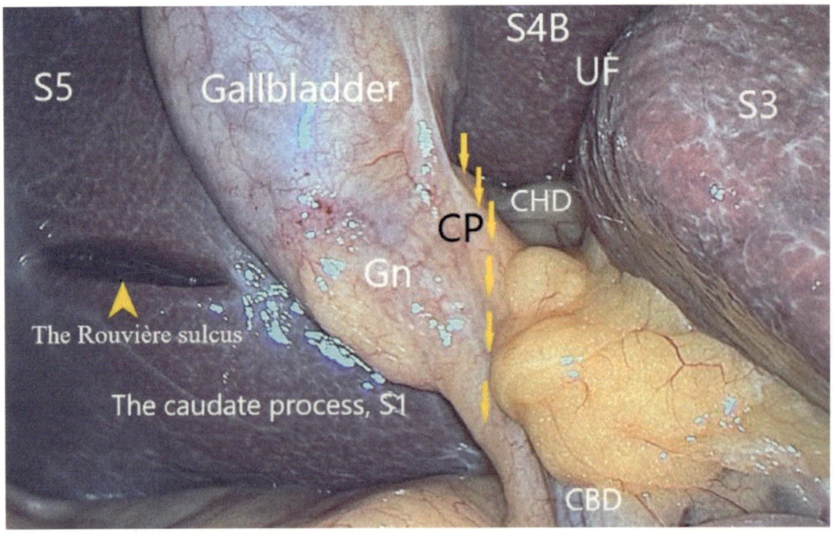

Figure 6.
Cystic pedicle: the anatomical site indicated by six arrows. Abbreviations: CP = cystic pedicle; Gn = gallbladder neck; CHD = common hepatic duct; CBD = common bile duct; S1 = the first liver segment; S3 = the third liver segment; UF = umbilical fissure; S4B = liver subsegment 4B; S5 = the fifth liver segment.

DOI: http://dx.doi.org/10.5772/intechopen.1011304

8.1 Cystic duct

The CD (*ductus cysticus*) is a part of the biliary ductal system. Typically measuring 2.5 cm in length, the CD can vary significantly, ranging from a few millimetres to 10 cm. It is typically 2.5 cm long, although variations exist, ranging from a few millimetres to 10 cm. The CD usually converges with the common hepatic duct 2–2.5 cm below the junction of the right and left hepatic ducts. The normal diameter of the CD is approximately 4.5 mm [30], with a lumen measuring 2–3 mm.

The mucosa of the CD resembles that of the Gn and contains 5–12 oblique folds known as spiral (Heister) valves. These folds contribute to the tortuosity of the CD and may promote the retention of small gallstones within the lumen. Additionally, the mucosa of the CD features a thin, incomplete muscle layer (*muscularis mucosae*), while its fibromuscular layer is structurally similar to that of the gallbladder. The proper muscularis layer is absent [69].

There are three common fusion patterns between the CD and common hepatic duct: angular, parallel, and spiral, with distributions of 75, 20, and 5%, respectively (**Figure 7**) [7]. The angle of fusion can range from a right angle to 10° [5]. In cases of spiral fusion, the CD may merge with the common hepatic duct at any point along its surface.

During cholecystectomy, an atypical fusion between the CD and the right hepatic (or sectional) bile duct should be recognised as a potential rare or very rare anatomical variation (**Figure 8**). Moreover, in sporadic cases, a small atypical bile duct may occasionally fuse with the CD.

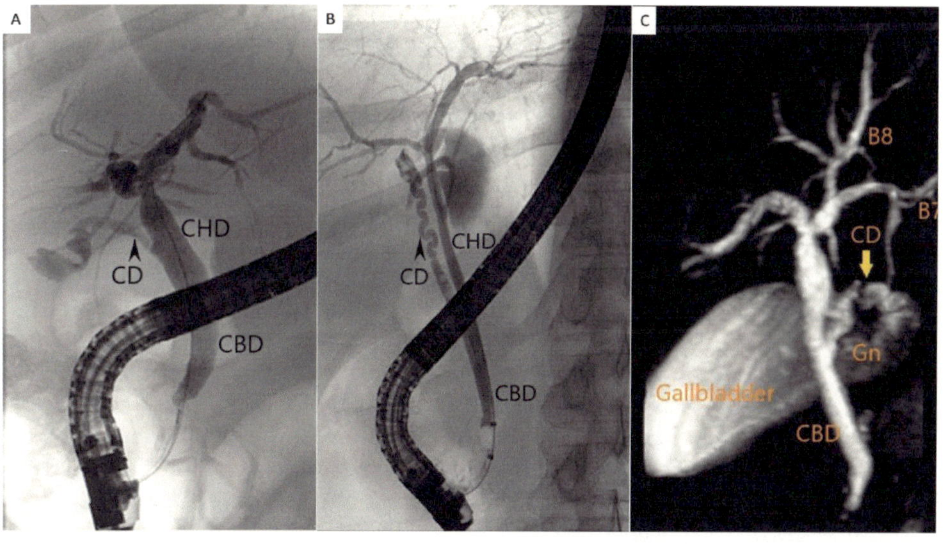

Figure 7.
The three most common patterns of fusion between the cystic duct and common hepatic duct are angular (A), parallel (B), and spiral (C). Small calculi are visible within the cystic duct, as shown in B. The retroductal spiral course of the cystic duct is shown in C. Abbreviations: CD = cystic duct; CHD = common hepatic duct; CBD = common bile duct; B7 = one of the bile ducts for liver segment 7; B8 = one of the bile ducts for liver segment 8.

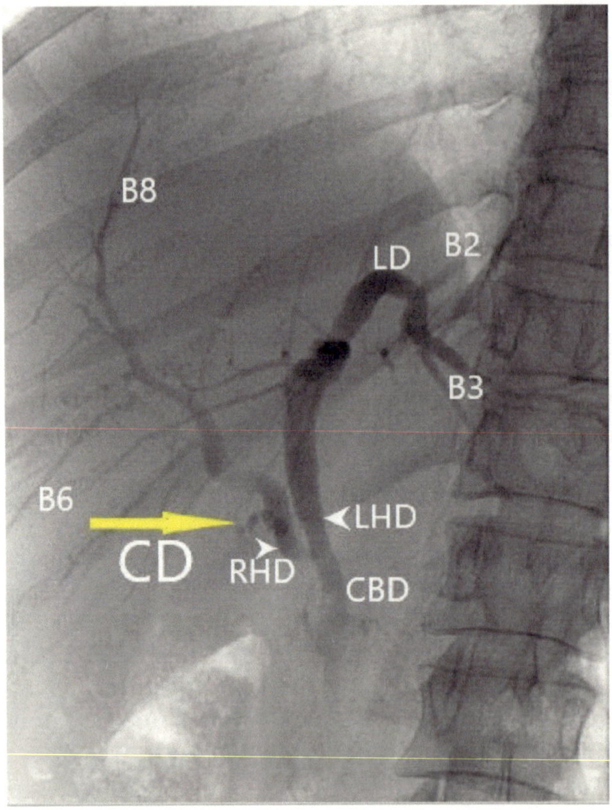

Figure 8.
Postoperative retrograde cholangiopancreatography: A rare anatomical variant. Cystic duct fusion with the right hepatic duct. Abbreviations: CD = cystic duct (arrow points at); RHD = right hepatic duct (arrow head points at); LHD = left hepatic duct (arrow head points at); CBD = common bile duct; LD = lateral duct (sectional); B2 = bile duct for liver segment 2; B3 = bile duct for liver segment 3; B6 = bile duct for liver segment 6; B8 = bile duct for liver segment 8.

8.2 Cystic artery

The cystic artery usually arises from the right hepatic artery and passes behind the common hepatic duct in 80% of the cases. Its average length is 2 cm. It is classified into three types based on length: short (<10 mm), typical (10–30 mm), and long (>30 mm). The diameter of the cystic artery is generally smaller than that of the CD.

The cystic artery is located on the cystic plate. The trunk of the cystic artery branches into superficial (anterior) and deep (posterior) branches. The superficial branch is often visible on the anterior surface of the peritoneal wall of the gallbladder (**Figure 9**), whereas the deep branch, which has a smaller diameter, runs behind the CD and emerges on the posterior part of the peritoneal wall of the gallbladder. In surgical practice, these are referred to as the medial and lateral branches of the cystic artery, respectively.

Variations in the systematic and topographical anatomy of the gallbladder arteries are common [70]. Two cystic arteries are found in 10% of individuals. A separate cystic artery located anterior to the CD strongly suggests that it originates from the proper hepatic artery. Other arteries, such as the middle hepatic artery, can also give rise to cystic arteries [70–72].

DOI: http://dx.doi.org/10.5772/intechopen.1011304

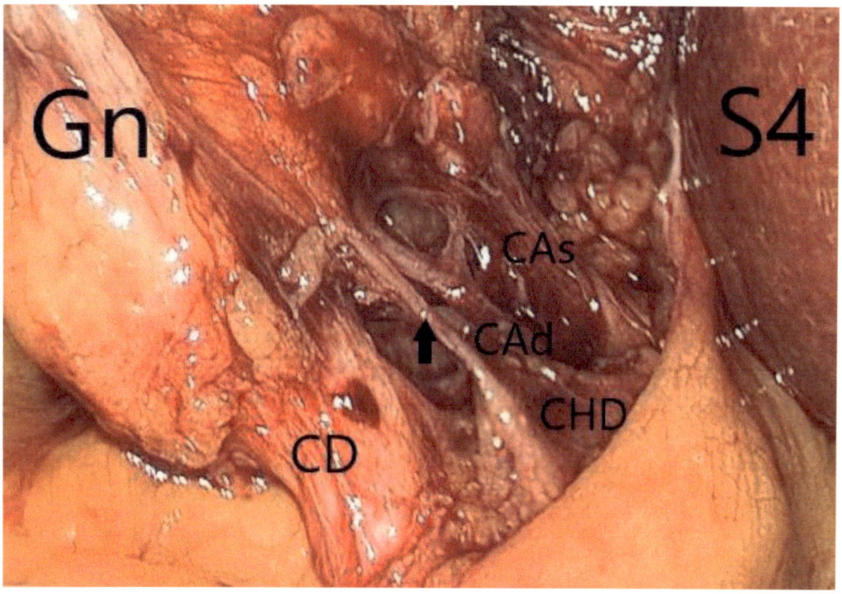

Figure 9.
Findings in the hepatocystic area during urgent laparoscopic cholecystectomy: Four tubular structures labelled as CAs, CAd, CD, and the one indicated by an arrow. Interpretation: The arrow indicates a tubular structure that may indicate a vessel or atypical bile duct. After further ablation of the hepatocystic area distally and posteriorly, each of the four tubular structures was clipped using medium-sized Weck Hem-o-lok polymer ligation clips. Abbreviations: CAs = superficial cystic artery (superficial branch of the cystic artery); CAd = deep cystic artery (deep branch of the cystic artery); CD = cystic duct; CHD = common hepatic duct; Gn = gallbladder neck; S4 = liver segment 4.

The main branches of the cystic artery further subdivide into finer branches within the outer layer of the SS, which then penetrate the inner SS layer.

8.3 Cystic veins

The Gf and Gb veins penetrate the liver parenchyma and drain directly into the hepatic venous system. These veins are often visible on the serosa of the peritoneal wall of the gallbladder.

There is no single constant venous trunk in the gallbladder. A small-diameter cystic vein, along with other veins from the common hepatic and bile ducts, drains into the portal vein. Occasionally, this vein can be observed within or behind Calot's triangle. During laparoscopic cholecystectomy, compression with metal or plastic clips may help prevent oozing.

8.4 Cystic lymph nodes

Numerous lymphatic vessels encircle the gallbladder and CD in the subserosal layers. During the infectious phase of acute cholecystitis, pathogens encounter the lymph node of Lund, which also serves as a sentinel node in gallbladder malignancies.

The Japanese lymph node classification categorises lymph nodes based on their anatomical location [45, 46]. It is a valuable tool for assessing carcinoma spread through the regional and distal lymph node systems (category 'N' of the TNM system). However, it can also help describe the locations of enlarged lymph nodes in patients with benign biliary diseases. For example, the lymph nodes surrounding the CD are classified as lymph node station 12c.

It is common to observe multiple cystic lymph nodes both within and outside the hepatocystic triangle (including in front of the CD) in cases of acute moderate Tokyo grade 2 cholecystitis [33, 73]. **Table 2** summarises the lymph nodes surrounding the gallbladder, extrahepatic ducts, and adjacent anatomical structures.

8.5 Cystic pedicle and the application of the critical view of the safety method

First, after incising the anterior serosa over the cystic pedicle at a safe location, usually below the lower Gb, the lateral margin of the cystic artery, or frequently the lateral margin of its superficial branch, serves as an anatomical landmark within the hepatocystic triangle. The first stage of surgery involves tunnelling and ablating the tissues of the SS-outer layer laterally between the artery and the lateral angle of the hepatocystic triangle [74]. The second stage involved exposing the CD to the

Station code	Substation	Group	Location
12	—	—	Hepatoduodenal ligament
	12a	—	Lymph nodes along the proper hepatic artery
	—	$12a_1$	Superior subgroup: it represents the cranial half located between the confluence of the right and left hepatic ducts and the upper border of the pancreas
	—	$12a_2$	Inferior subgroup: it is a caudal half between the confluence of the right and left hepatic ducts and the upper border of the pancreas
	12b	—	Lymph nodes along the bile duct
	—	$12b_1$	Superior subgroup: lymph nodes on the anterior, posterior, and right side surfaces of the bile duct in the cranial half between the confluence of the right and left hepatic ducts and the upper border of the pancreas
	—	$12b_2$	Inferior subgroup: lymph nodes on the anterior, posterior, and right side surfaces of the bile duct in the caudal half between the confluence of the right and left hepatic ducts and the upper border of the pancreas
	12c	—	Lymph nodes around the cystic duct
	12 h	—	Lymph nodes in the hepatic side of the confluence of the right and left hepatic duct
	12p	—	Lymph nodes posterior to portal vein
	—	$12p_1$	Superior subgroup: it is a posterior surface of the portal vein in the cranial half between the confluence of the right and left hepatic ducts and the upper border of the pancreas
	—	$12p_2$	Inferior subgroup: it is a posterior surface of the portal vein in the caudal half between the confluence of the right and left hepatic ducts and the upper border of the pancreas
13	—	—	Lymph nodes on the posterior surface of the head of the pancreas
	13a	—	Superior subgroup: lymph nodes cranial to the duodenal papilla
	13b	—	Inferior subgroup: lymph nodes caudal to the duodenal papilla

Table 2.
Classification of regional lymph node stations No. 12 and No. 13 and their anatomical location [45, 46].

DOI: http://dx.doi.org/10.5772/intechopen.1011304

surrounding subserosal tissues. Finally, the third stage requires complete or near-complete skeletonisation of the cystic artery or its branches as close as possible to the hepatic wall of the gallbladder.

Second, precise identification of the cystic artery and duct during laparoscopic cholecystectomy requires sufficient ablation of the hepatocystic area. Theoretically, tissues should be ablated from the surface of one-third of the hepatic wall of the gallbladder (**Figure 10**) [74]. However, caution must be exercised in this approach, as the extent of hepatic wall exposure is often limited by biliary pathology, such as significant changes in the cross-sectional structure of the gallbladder wall. In acute surgical cases, exposure is often less than one-third (typically, 20–25%). Attempting to separate the hepatic wall of the gallbladder from the SS-outer layer in these circumstances poses a high risk of bleeding or injury to the extrahepatic bile ducts.

Third, the superficial branch of the cystic artery is sometimes mistaken for the main trunk. A thinner deep branch and/or its second-order branches are typically divided using electrocautery within the SS-outer layer. However, unexpected bleeding from the deep branch of the cystic artery poses a significant clinical challenge.

Fourth, clinically significant bleeding from the superficial branch of the cystic artery may occur during subtotal cholecystectomy. In contrast, bleeding from a deep branch of the cystic artery on the lateral side of the peritoneal wall of the gallbladder is uncommon.

Fifth, a large or moderately sized gallstone lodged in the Gn for an extended period can exert pressure on the gallbladder wall within Calot's triangle. Over time, the walls of the gallbladder and common duct in contact undergo gradual atrophy due to secondary intramural chronic ischaemic changes [75]. Surgical manipulation to expose the SS-inner layer, Calot, or hepatocystic triangles during this stage of gallstone disease is risky. In such cases, STC is considered a safer alternative.

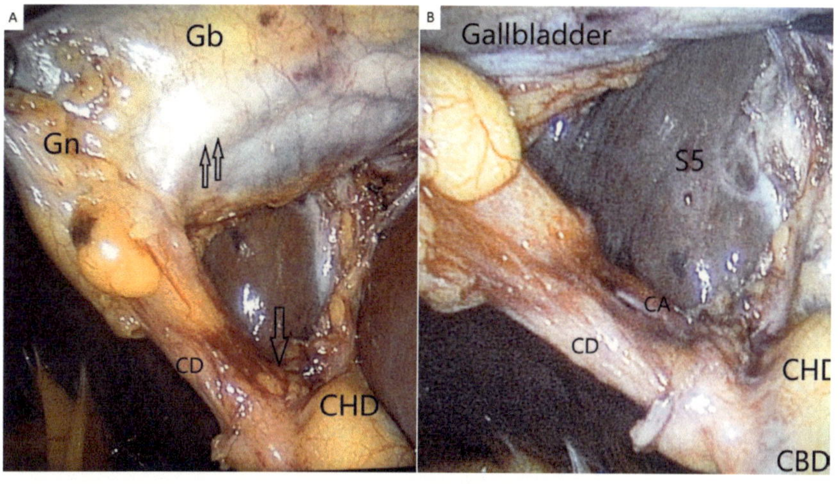

Figure 10.
Laparoscopic cholecystectomy: the hepatocystic area comprises one-third of the hepatic wall of the gallbladder. A: A single arrow indicates a potential site for the cystic artery between the cystic duct and the common hepatic duct. Two smaller arrows indicate the longitudinal deformity of the anterior part of the peritoneal wall, which is a superficial branch of the cystic artery. B: The cystic artery separated from the cystic duct; narrow Calot's triangle exposed. Abbreviations: Gb = gallbladder body; Gn = gallbladder neck; CD = cystic duct; CHD = common hepatic duct; CBD = common bile duct; S5 = liver segment 5.

9. The cystic plate as a component of the hepatic plate and liver-gate theory

9.1 The concept of the hepatic plate

The hepatic plate system consists of four interconnected connective tissue plates: the hilar plate (central part), cystic plate (right lateral side), umbilical plate (left anterolateral side), and Arantian plate (left posterolateral side). Histologically, the hepatic plate and Glissonian sheaths are identical structures [26, 49, 50, 76, 77]. A narrow gap exists between the cystic plate and Laënnec's capsule, forming an anatomical plane for five-layer cystic plate cholecystectomy, which may be performed independently or as an adjunct to resectional hepatobiliary surgery [49].

9.2 Liver-gate theory

There are two strategies for accessing the Glissonian pedicles for anatomical liver resection: intrafascial (intraglissonian) and extrafascial (Glissonian approach). The latter is based on the 'liver-gate theory', which is crucial for resecting liver sections, segments, and subsegments (cone units). According to this concept, the Glissonian pedicles of these anatomical units can only be safely accessed and surgically isolated between Laënnec's capsule (serving as a landmark) and the Glissonian sheaths (the target) at six specific locations, without necessitating liver parenchymal transection. These six locations are referred to as the liver gates or gates of the liver. They are positioned between four anatomical landmarks on the inferior surface of the liver: the Arantius plate, umbilical plate, cystic plate, and caudate process pedicle (G1c) [26, 49, 50, 78–81].

Surgical extrahepatic dissection between two neighbouring liver gates provides an entry point into the space between Laënnec's capsule and the second-order Glissonian pedicles, allowing for extrahepatic exposure, encirclement, and isolation of the sectional Glissonian pedicles without damaging the surrounding liver parenchyma. Limited liver transection may be permissible to avoid injury to the sectional and segmental Glissonian pedicles. This manoeuvre aims to control the inflow to the sections of the hemiliver before parenchymal transection.

The Takasaki approach involves extrahepatic encirclement of the anterior Glissonian pedicle (Gant) and posterior Glissonian pedicle (Gpost) using the right-sided liver gates IV, V, and VI [78, 79]. The Gant is accessible by detaching the cystic plate from Laënnec's capsule in a procedure called 'cystic plate cholecystectomy', which connects Gates IV and V. Once the cystic plate cholecystectomy is completed, Gpost can be isolated by connecting Gates V and VI. The left-sided sectional pedicles can be accessed through Gates I, II, and III. **Table 3** provides topographic descriptions of the liver gates [26, 49, 50, 81].

According to the six-layer gallbladder wall theory, the cystic plate represents the fifth layer of the gallbladder hepatic wall. Anatomically, the medial portion of the cystic plate encircles both the Gant and Gpost. The most medial area of the cystic plate, where it connects with the hilar plate, forms Gate IV in the liver.

The hepatic plate concept and liver-gate theory serve as a reminder to gallbladder surgeons that the area behind the medial portion of the hepatic wall of the gallbladder and the medial part of the hepatocystic region is a high risk zone, containing right-sided Glissonian pedicles between liver gates. This zone of danger poses significant challenges during biliary surgery, particularly in cases of a small, severely contracted

DOI: http://dx.doi.org/10.5772/intechopen.1011304

Gates	Location
I	Juncture between the Arantius and the umbilical plates: above G1 and the Arantius ligament.
II	Juncture between the round liver ligament and the umbilical plate, which can be approached by dividing the falciform ligament at the level of the liver surface.
III	Juncture between the hilar plate and the right side of the umbilical plate; the site of the right edge of the Glissonian pedicle and root of the umbilical portion—Gup (G2 + G3 + G4): to the right of the falciform ligament and above the hilar plate.
IV	Juncture of the left (medial) portion of the cystic plate and the hilar plate. It is above and behind the right anterior portal vein. The left portion of the cystic plate is also referred to as the post-cystic pedicle, the lower proximal point of the cystic plate, or the left edge of the posterior extremity of the cystic plate for the anterior Glissonian pedicle.
V	The hepatic hilum area between the bifurcation of anterior/posterior Glissonian pedicles and the right main Glissonian pedicle.
VI	The space between the posterior Glissonian pedicle and the G1c.

Abbreviations: G1 = Glissonian pedicle for liver segment 1; Gup = Glissonian pedicles at the root of the umbilical portion; G2 = Glissonian pedicle for liver segment 2; G3 = Glissonian pedicle for liver segment 3; G4 = Glissonian pedicle for liver segment 4; G1c = Glissonian pedicle for caudate process of liver segment 1.

Table 3.
Extrahepatic gates to the liver and topographical characterisation of six interfaces between Laënnec's capsule and Glissonian pedicles.

gallbladder or severely damaged intrahepatic gallbladder. In such scenarios, the three requirements of the critical view of safety theory [74] should not be applied [80].

9.3 Conventional cholecystectomy viewed through the lens of the hepatic plate concept and liver-gate theory

First, exposure of the liver parenchyma or bleeding from the liver during a conventional three-layer cholecystectomy indicates full-thickness surgical injury to the cystic plate and Laënnec's capsule. Second, the supravesical (or subvesical/Luschka) bile ducts do not fuse with the gallbladder cavity; rather, they are separated by Laënnec's capsule and/or the cystic plate. Bile leakage from these ducts occurs due to a full-thickness injury to the cystic plate and, in some cases, Laënnec's capsule, during conventional cholecystectomy. The classification of bile duct injuries, particularly those related to supravesical (peripheral) bile duct injuries, requires attention [82, 83].

Third, when a severely inflamed gallbladder is evident or suspected to be adhering to the right-sided Glissonian pedicles, an immediate bailout surgical procedure must be considered.

Fourth, G1c is identified at the medial entry of the well-contoured Rouvière sulcus. If the Rouvière sulcus is short, G1c may be observed at a distance from the sulcus, representing a non-touch zone for gallbladder surgeons.

Fifth, the cystic plate serves as a landmark for the inferior edge in a total five-layer cholecystectomy, which is indicated when gallbladder cancer is suspected. Six conditions fall under the category of 'suspected gallbladder cancer': elevated lesions >10 mm in diameter; increasing tumour size compared to previous radiological findings; sessile lesions; irregular wall thickness lesions that mimic cancer; elevated lesions with dense enhancement; and positive accumulation on fluorodeoxyglucose positron emission tomography (FDG PET), defined as an 18F-FDG maximum standardised uptake value >3.65 [76]. Further treatment options depend on the histological examination of the resected gallbladder. The term '*whole-layer cholecystectomy*' is used in surgical practice as an alternative to '*five-layer cholecystectomy*'.

10. Main bile duct

10.1 Anatomy

The term '*common duct*' in textbooks refers to two bile ducts: the common hepatic duct and the common bile duct. However, the alternative term '*main bile duct*' provides greater clarity when the anatomical classification of the common duct does not apply. This terminology is particularly useful in contexts such as reporting radiological findings when the CD is unidentifiable, as well as in the diagnosis and surgery of gallbladder or bile duct cancer [84]. Describing abnormalities of the main bile duct using the system of thirds— upper, middle, and lower third—is a recognised and accepted method [45, 46, 85].

10.1.1 Common hepatic duct

The common hepatic duct (*ductus hepaticus communis*) is formed at the junction of the right and left hepatic ducts. It typically measures 2–2.5 cm when the fusion pattern of the cystic and common hepatic ducts is angular. However, depending on the location of the junction with the CD, its length can vary from 1 to 10 cm.

10.1.2 Common bile duct

The common bile duct (*ductus choledochus*) measures 7.5–10 cm in length. It is formed by the junction of the CD and common hepatic ducts. Its anatomical topography is characterised by its relationship with the duodenum. The common bile duct consists of four portions: supraduodenal, retroduodenal, infraduodenal (intrapancreatic), and intraduodenal [2, 6].

The supraduodenal portion (*pars supraduodenalis*) is approximately 2.5–3 cm long and runs along the right side of the hepatoduodenal ligament. The section of the common bile duct situated between the superior margin of the duodenum (*bulbus duodeni* or D1) and the head of the pancreas (*caput pancreatis*) is known as the retroduodenal portion (*pars retroduodenalis*). Three vessels—the gastroduodenal artery (*arteria gastroduodenalis*) on the left side, the posterior superior pancreaticoduodenal artery (*arteria pancreaticoduodenal superior posterior*) anteriorly, and the portal vein (*vena portae hepatis*) posteriorly—encircle this section of the common bile duct. This anatomical relationship between the common bile duct and surrounding vascular structures should be considered during emergency laparotomy for bleeding from a posterior duodenal ulcer.

The infraduodenal (intrapancreatic) portion (*pars infraduodenalis; pars intrapancreatica*) typically resides in a groove, although it may occasionally be enclosed within a tunnel of the pancreatic head, surrounded by the vascular arcades between the superior and inferior pancreaticoduodenal arteries. The most distal section of the common bile duct, the intraduodenal part (*pars intraduodenalis*), traverses the wall of the second part of the duodenum at an oblique angle, where it merges with the pancreatic duct (*ductus pancreaticus*), also known as the duct of Wirsung, forming the hepatopancreatic ampulla. This structure, along with the surrounding sphincter of Oddi, contributes to the formation of the greater duodenal papilla (*papilla Vateri*), located in the posterior wall of the duodenum. This anatomical arrangement of the infraduodenal portion of the common bile duct is observed in two-thirds of patients [86–88].

Similar to other bile ducts, the common bile duct lacks peristaltic contractile activity and primarily functions as a conduit for bile transport to the duodenum. The standard diameter of the common duct is ≤6 mm, typically ranging between 4 and 6 mm. A diameter of ≥7 mm is a cause for concern and requires further investigation.

10.2 Histology

Most bile ducts consist of a columnar epithelium, basement membrane, subepithelial layer, and fibrotic layer. Similar to the CD, the common bile duct has a thin and incomplete muscularis mucosa. Another histological characteristic of the biliary ductal system is the presence of mucous glands distributed along both the intrahepatic and extrahepatic bile ducts. These glands are particularly prominent in the distal portion of the common bile duct.

10.3 Inspection during open and laparoscopic cholecystectomy

First, the common hepatic duct, its junction with the CD, and the supraduodenal section of the common bile duct are the biliary structures that should be identified before transecting the CD during an open cholecystectomy. Notably, the proper hepatic artery may be positioned in front of the common and cystic bile ducts when originating from the superior mesenteric or gastroduodenal arteries. This variation occurs in one out of every 10–20 patients.

Second, the hepatoduodenal ligament must be inspected during the initial phase of laparoscopic cholecystectomy [88]. Common hepatic and bile ducts are often observed, particularly in elective surgical settings. In these instances, the common duct (not the imaginary lines) serves as the primary anatomical landmark for safe laparoscopic cholecystectomy.

11. First-, second-, and third-order division bile ducts

Figure 11 illustrates the classified bile ducts, excluding those associated with liver segment 1. The right and left hepatic ducts are designated as first-order division bile ducts. Sectional bile ducts (anterior, posterior, medial, and lateral) are categorised as second-order division bile ducts. The segmental bile ducts B2, B3, B4, B5, B6, B7, and B8 are identified as third-order division bile ducts. This classification of the bile ducts fully aligns with the anatomical units of the liver defined by the portal vein rami, which are hierarchically organised as follows: the hemiliver as the first-order liver division, the section as the second-order division, and the segment as the third-order division [10–12, 45].

Figure 12 illustrates a unique case of biliary anatomy. This highlights the significance of non-invasive preoperative imaging techniques for the biliary system, such as computed tomography cholangiography or magnetic resonance imaging cholangiography, in patients awaiting cholecystectomy.

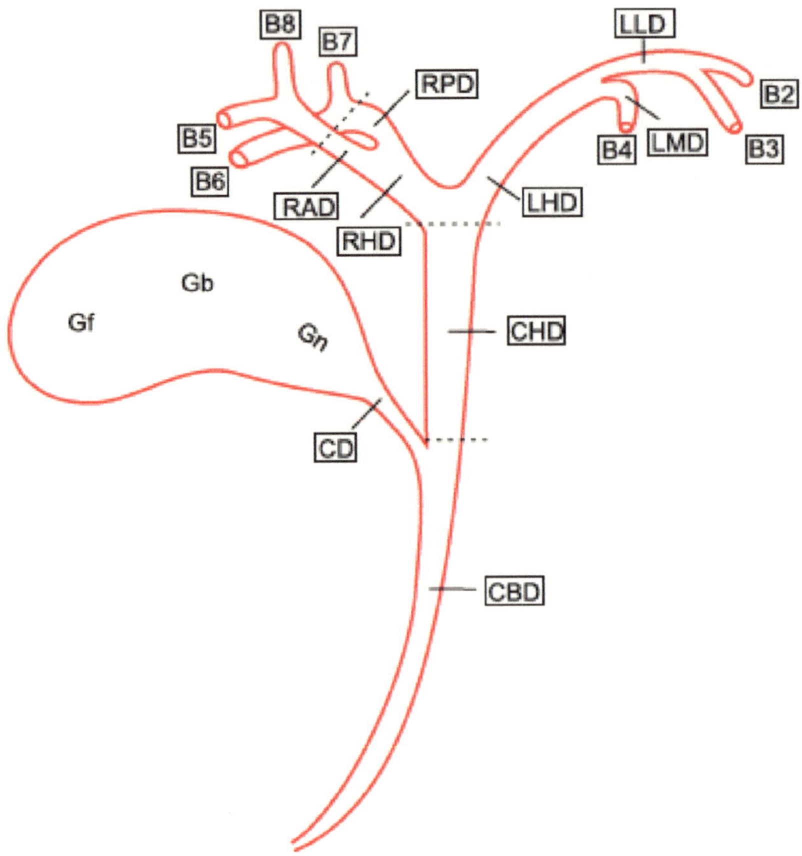

Figure 11.
The scheme of the extrahepatic biliary system (excluding the bile ducts of liver segment 1, which are described in **Table 4***). Abbreviations: B = segmental bile duct (B2, B3, B4, B5, B6, B7, B8); RAD = right anterior duct (sectional); RPD = right posterior duct (sectional); LLD = left lateral duct (sectional); LMD = left medial duct (sectional); RHD = right hepatic duct (for right hemiliver); LHD = left hepatic duct (for left hemiliver); CHD = common hepatic duct; Gf = gallbladder fundus; Gb = gallbladder body; Gn = gallbladder neck; CD = cystic duct; CBD = common bile duct.*

12. Fourth-order division and the bile ducts for liver segment 1

A subsegment of the liver is an anatomical part of the Couinaud segment consisting of either a single conical unit or, more commonly, a group of such units, each defined by its subsegmental portal inflow [78, 92]. It represents a fourth-order division of the liver territory and is the smallest classification level within the anatomical hierarchy based on the portal vein ramifications.

The patterns of the liver subsegmental structures vary within each segment. However, the basic fourth-order division patterns for segments S1, S4, and S8 are widely recognised. The Spiegel, paracaval, and caudate subsegments of S1; apical (cranial or superior) and basal (caudal or inferior, as defined by Healey and Schroy [3]) subsegments of S4; and ventral and dorsal subsegments of S8 are consistent anatomical units of the liver. Each of these units has a distinct portal inflow and biliary ductal systems. Notably, variations in the subsegmental structures are common, even within these three segments. Such variations are integral to the classification of fourth-order division bile ducts [53, 89, 90]. **Figure 13** provides a summary of these

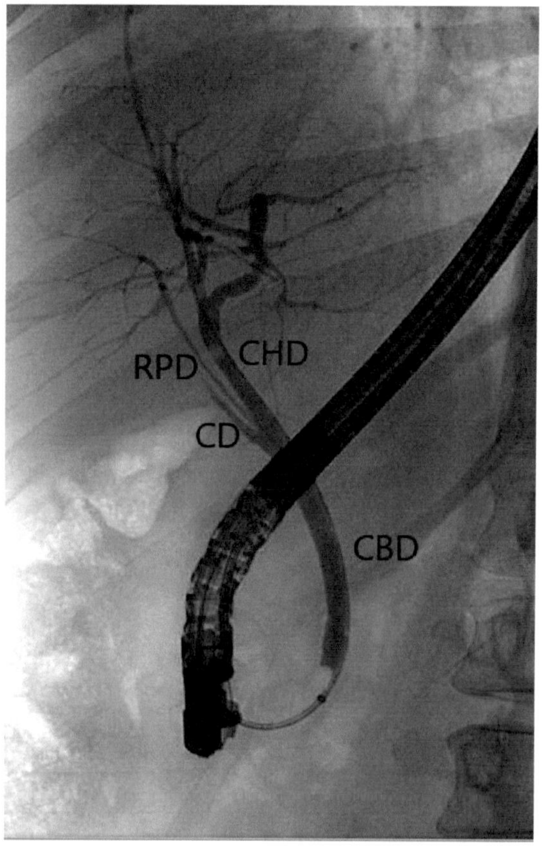

Figure 12.
A two-dimensional endoscopic cholangiopancreatography image illustrates the unusual anatomy of the posterior duct, which is located between the cystic duct and the common hepatic duct. This area corresponds to the hepatocystic and Calot's triangles. Obstructive jaundice due to cholangiolithiasis served as the indication for therapeutic endoscopic cholangiopancreatography. A laparoscopic STC-2A open-tract subtotal cholecystectomy (Section 14.2) was performed for acute suppurative calculous cholecystitis during emergency admission a few weeks later. Abbreviations: CD = cystic duct; RPD = right posterior duct; CHD = common hepatic duct; CBD = common bile duct.

basic anatomical relationships. **Table 4** provides additional details on the subsegmental nomenclature of the liver and its pedicles [53, 89–91].

The five subsegmental bile ducts of the first liver segment—B1li, B1ls, B1r1, B1r2, and B1c—are exceptions to the standard nomenclature as they drain into three bile ducts: B1li and B1ls converge with the left hepatic duct, B1r1 and B1r2 merge with the posterior bile duct, and B1c joins the right hepatic duct (**Table 4**). **Figure 14** illustrates the view behind the gallbladder after lifting the neck during laparoscopic surgery. This manoeuvre exposes the Glissonian pedicle connected to the caudate process of the liver.

This anatomical concept is essential for liver resection. For example, performing anatomical segmentectomy or subsegmentectomy is not feasible without the Glissonian approach, selective inflow clamping with or without indigo carmine or methylene blue dye injection into the corresponding portal vein (positive staining effect), and/or systematic indocyanine green (ICG) injection after selective inflow clamping (negative staining effect) [92].

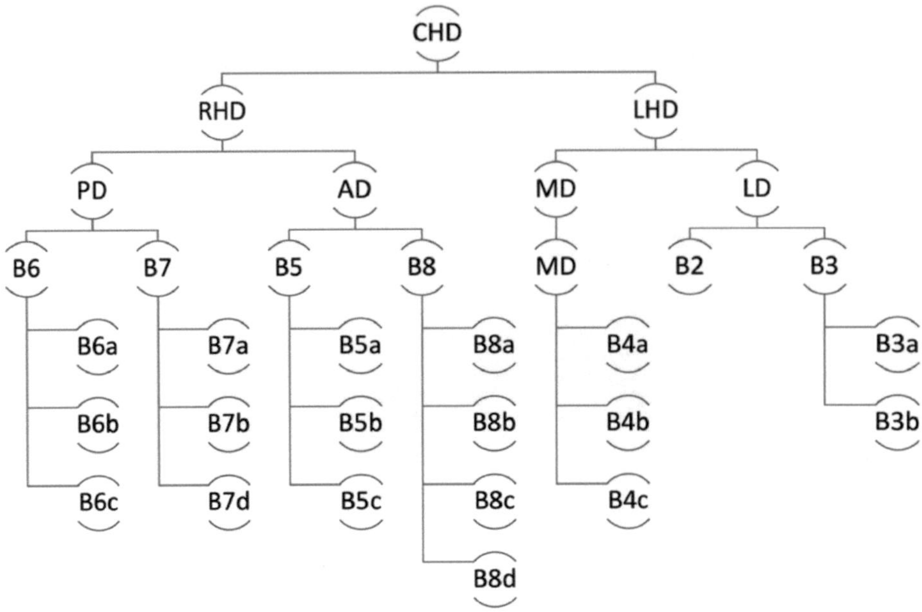

Figure 13.
Hierarchy chart of the bile ducts based on their four-stage order, from the first to the fourth. Numbers indicate Couinaud's segments, and the lowercase letters denote subsegments. Abbreviations: CHD = common hepatic duct; RHD = right hepatic duct; LHD = left hepatic duct; PD = posterior duct; AD = anterior duct; MD = medial duct; LD = lateral duct; B = bile duct.

Couinaud's segment	Subsegment (cone unit)	Glissonian pedicle	Bile duct	Comments on subsegmental duct branches and the alternative terms
S1	S1li: left inferior	G1li	B1li	For Spiegel's lobe
	S1ls: left superior	G1ls	B1ls	For Spiegel's lobe
	S1r1: right 1	G1r1	B1r1	For paracaval portion
	S1r2: right 2	G1r2	B1r2	For paracaval portion
	S1c: caudate process	G1c	B1c	For caudate process
S2	—	G2	B2	—
S3	S3a: superior	G3a	B3a	B3s/G3s: superior
	S3b: inferior	G3b	B3b	B3i/G3i inferior
S4	S4a: superior	G4a	B4a	B4s/G4: apical; cranial
	S4b: inferior	G4b	B4b	B4i/G4i: basal; caudal
	S4c: dorsal; middle cranial	G4c	B4c	B4d/G4d: dorsal; middle cranial
S5	S5a: ventral	G5a	B5a	B5v/G5v: ventral
	S5b: dorsal	G5b	B5b	B5d/G5d: dorsal
	S5c: lateral	G5c	B5c	B5l/G5l: lateral
S6	S6a: ventral	G6a	B6a	B6vG6v: ventral

Couinaud's segment	Subsegment (cone unit)	Glissonian pedicle	Bile duct	Comments on subsegmental duct branches and the alternative terms
	S6b: dorsal	G6b	B6b	B6d/G6d: dorsal
	S6c: lateral	G6c	B6c	B6l/G6l: lateral
S7	S7a: ventral	G7a	B7a	B7v/G7v: ventral
	S7b: dorsal	G7b	B7b	B7d/G7d: dorsal
	S7d: medial	G7d	B7d	B7m/G7m: medial
S8	S8a: ventral	G8a	B8a	B8v/G8v: ventral
	S8b: lateral	G8b	B8b	B8l/G8l: lateral
	S8c: dorsal	G8c	B8c	B8d/G8d: dorsal
	S8d: medial	G8d	B8d	B8m/G8m: medial

Numbers refer to Couinaud's segments, except for r1 and r2. The paracaval portion is part of liver S1 (not Segment 9). The nomenclature for the subsegmental structures li, ls, r1, r2, 1c, a, b, c, and d is based on the Nagoya subsegmental bile duct classification [53, 89, 90]. The alternative subsegmental nomenclature [91] is presented in column 5: i (inferior), s (superior), v (ventral), d (dorsal), l (lateral), and m (medial). The term 'cone unit' is an alternative term for 'subsegment' [92]. The adjectives attributed to S4—apical, caudal, middle, and cranial—were used in the Precision Anatomy for Minimally Invasive Hepatopancreatobiliary Surgery (PAM-HPB) Consensus 2020 meeting [92]. Other abbreviations: S = liver segment; B = bile duct; G = Glissonian pedicle; li = left inferior; ls = left superior; r = right; 1c = caudate process.

Table 4.
The list of liver subsegments (cone units), Glissonian pedicles, and bile ducts is organised according to their topography within the segment.

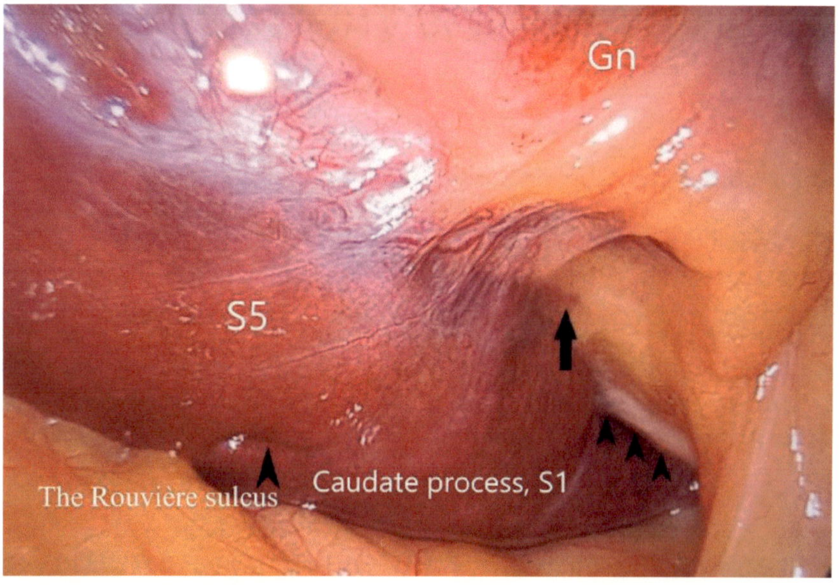

Figure 14.
The posterior wall of the gallbladder neck and the cystic pedicle are displayed. The three arrowheads indicate a structure linked to the caudate process of liver segment 1, Glissonian pedicle 1C. The arrow above the three arrowheads marks the location corresponding to the posterior Glissonian pedicle (posterior duct). Abbreviations: S1 = liver segment 1; S5 = liver segment 5.

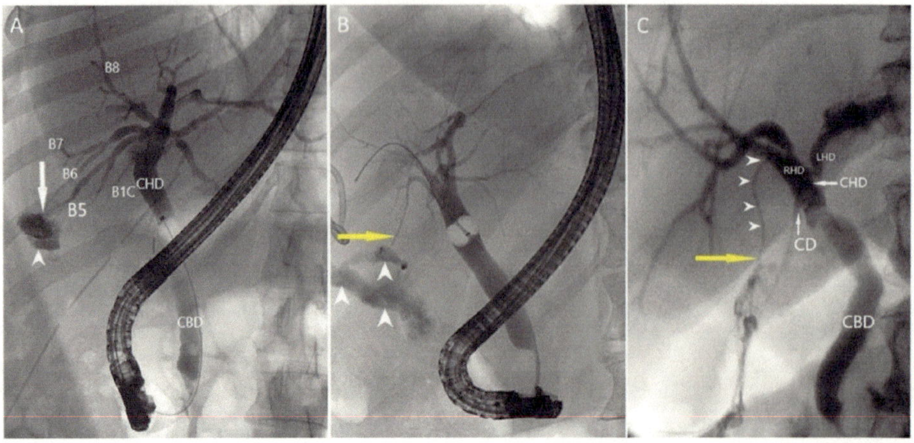

Figure 15.
Injured peripheral bile ducts. A: The subsegmental bile duct of segment 5; the white arrow points to the leaking bile duct, and the arrowhead indicates the collection of contrast material used for endoscopic retrograde cholangiography. B: Similar findings are observed in a different patient. C: Similar findings in a different patient; note the injured and leaking bile duct B5, laterally from the serosa of the gallbladder mid-body; four arrowheads indicate its course; it fuses with a sectional bile duct. Abbreviations: B5, B6, B7, B8, and B1C = bile ducts of liver segments 5, 6, 7, 8, and caudate process of segment 1; CD = cystic duct; RHD = right hepatic duct; LHD = left hepatic duct; CHD = common hepatic duct; CBD = common bile duct.

A detailed understanding of this anatomy is important for gallbladder and bile duct surgeons. Precise descriptions of unexpected complications, such as biliary leaks from peripheral ducts in liver segments S5 and S4 or subsegment 1C (caudate process), are crucial during and after the cholecystectomy. **Figure 15** presents the findings related to these complications.

13. Anchors and other Glissonian pedicles

An anchor is a technical term referring to thin, cord-like, or membrane-like structures frequently located at the orifices of Glissonian pedicles. They connect the pedicles to Laënnec's capsule. Anchors typically surround sectional Glissonian pedicles, such as Gant and Gpost, and segmental pedicles, such as G4. In some cases, they may also contain a bile duct (**Figure 16A**). Anatomical structures resembling anchors can also be found around the gallbladder. However, these are generally associated with the sectional anterior or posterior bile ducts (**Figure 16B**). During liver resection, careful dissection, isolation, ligation, and division of these anatomical structures are necessary to prevent bile leakage [79].

Superficial Glissonian pedicles with large bile ducts surrounding the gallbladder on both the superior and inferior liver surfaces are uncommon. Nevertheless, intra-operative scenarios demonstrating their presence have been documented (**Figure 17**). When performing cholecystectomy, meticulous use of diathermy is essential to avoid accidental contact with the liver serosa, thereby preventing injury to the bile ducts or parenchymal bleeding.

DOI: http://dx.doi.org/10.5772/intechopen.1011304

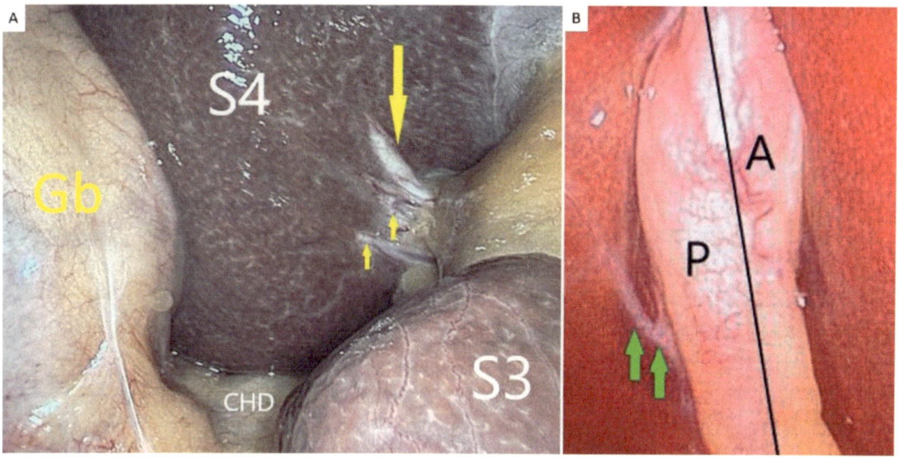

Figure 16.
Anchors. A: A large arrow and two smaller arrows indicate the biliary structures connecting liver segment S4 to other ducts located within the umbilical fissure of the liver. B: Green arrows denote a tubular structure (Glissonian, biliary) positioned behind the posterior surface of the peritoneal wall of the gallbladder, which is not connected to the gallbladder. Abbreviations: Gb = gallbladder body; CHD = common hepatic duct; S4 = the fourth liver segment; S3 = the third liver segment; P = posterior part of the peritoneal wall of the gallbladder; A = anterior part of the peritoneal wall of the gallbladder.

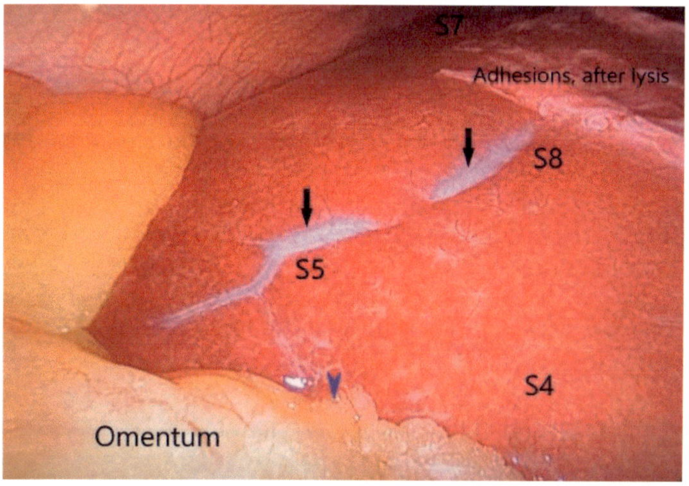

Figure 17.
Subcapsular Glissonian pedicles are located on the superior surface of the anterior section of the right hemiliver. The visible structures resemble bile ducts, as indicated by the two arrows. A blue arrowhead indicates the site of the gallbladder fundus, which is obscured by the greater omentum. The abbreviations S4, S5, S7, and S8 denote the liver segments.

14. Types of cholecystectomies

Two structural criteria define the type of cholecystectomy: the dissecting layer of the hepatic wall of the gallbladder and the completeness of gallbladder resection.

Other classifications of cholecystectomy are based on factors unrelated to the anatomical structure of the gallbladder. One such classification differentiates between open and laparoscopic cholecystectomy, with or without the use of robotic devices, depending on the surgical approach and technological adjuncts employed in the gallbladder surgery. Regarding the surgical setting, cholecystectomies, like all surgical procedures, can be categorised into two broad types: elective (planned) and emergency (unplanned). Furthermore, country-specific classifications are used to categorise surgical procedures by urgency, including cholecystectomy. The National Confidential Enquiry into Patient Outcome and Deathclassification of interventions has been used in England, Wales, Northern Ireland, and the Offshore British Islands [93]. This system classifies surgical procedures into four urgency levels: immediate, urgent, expedited, and elective.

14.1 Cholecystectomy classification based on the dissecting layer

This classification is based on the six-layer gallbladder theory. It includes three types of cholecystectomy: conventional (three-layer), cystic plate (five-layer), and full-thickness (six-layer) cholecystectomy.

First, conventional or three-layer cholecystectomy involves complete excision of the gallbladder between the inner and outer layers of the SS. In terms of the classical structure of the gallbladder wall, this is referred to as a two-layer (mucosa and fibromuscular) cholecystectomy because the separation plane passes through the alveolar tissue of the adventitia. Benign gallbladder disease is an indication for three-layer cholecystectomy.

Second, cystic plate cholecystectomy is a five-layer procedure, with the tissue separation plane lying in the small space between Laënnec's capsule and the cystic plate, specifically between the fifth and sixth layers of the hepatic wall of the gallbladder. The steps for this procedure are as follows [49]:

1. A circumferential incision is made in the serosa between the liver and gallbladder.

2. The space between Laënnec's capsule and the cystic plate at the junction of Gb and Gn are identified.

3. The gallbladder from Laënnec's capsule is separated, with the option of using tape to secure the gallbladder between Laënnec's capsule and the cystic plate.

4. Bluntly dissecting the gallbladder from Laënnec's capsule toward the Gf, taking care to avoid peeling off Laënnec's capsule, which may cause bleeding from the liver parenchyma.

5. Cholecystectomy is performed if this is the objective of the surgery. Six indications (under the term 'suspected gallbladder cancer') for cystic plate cholecystectomy are discussed in Section 9.3 [76].

6. When cystic plate cholecystectomy is part of anatomical liver resection, it involves methodical exposure and access to sectional Glissonian pedicles (as detailed in Sections 9.1 and 9.2). This technique is considered the standard manoeuvre for isolating the extrahepatic Gant pedicle.

Third, full-thickness or six-layer cholecystectomy involves the excision of Laënnec's capsule, which may be bluntly detached from the liver parenchyma. Laparoscopic full-thickness cholecystectomy is indicated for early-stage gallbladder cancer without liver invasion. However, if imaging reveals an ill-defined border between the gallbladder lesion and liver parenchyma, a laparoscopic full-thickness cholecystectomy with resection of 1–2 cm of the surrounding liver parenchyma is recommended. A thorough histological assessment of excised tissue is essential for planning further treatment in patients diagnosed with gallbladder cancer [76]. Therefore, a six-layer cholecystectomy is also referred to as biopsy cholecystectomy. The laparoscopic approach is preferable when biopsy cholecystectomy is the intended surgical outcome.

Alternative terms for five- and six-layer cholecystectomies include whole-layer cholecystectomy or laparoscopic whole-layer cholecystectomy [14, 76] and gallbladder bed dissection or laparoscopic gallbladder bed dissection [76].

14.1.1 Surgical strategies for identifying the CD and cystic artery during laparoscopic cholecystectomy

There are two primary surgical strategies for identifying the CD and cystic artery: the '*infundibular view*' and the '*critical view of safety*'. These are often referred to as methods.

The infundibular method involves identifying the CD, the junction between the CD and Gn, and a 5–7 mm segment of the Gn. This segment of the extrahepatic biliary system is known as the infundibulum, which is a crucial part of the gallbladder-CD complex for safe laparoscopic cholecystectomy. In this method, the CD is obstructed (using clips) and divided. Definitive exposure, clipping, and division of the cystic artery constitute the second surgical stage of this method. Therefore, Calot's triangle is the principal focus of '*infundibular*' laparoscopic cholecystectomies. The inability to isolate the '*infundibulum*' indicates the need to convert from laparoscopic surgery to laparotomy for complete cholecystectomy. It should also be noted that STC, a surgical option for challenging anatomical situations, was well-known (although not universally recognised) in the 1990s and earlier [94].

The '*critical view of safety*' method involves exposing and identifying both the cystic artery and duct before clipping and dividing them. A key condition for achieving this view of safety is to separate the CD and proximal third of the gallbladder from the surrounding pericholecystic connective tissue. The working area for this technique, comprising one-third of the hepatic wall of the gallbladder, is known as the hepatocystic triangle.

Although the '*critical view of safety*' is a widely accepted strategy in laparoscopic cholecystectomy, it is important to note that the theory behind this method does not specify how to achieve this view. In other words, tactical intraoperative decision-making is left to the surgeon, who relies entirely on practical experience and prevailing practices of their surgical training.

The effectiveness of the 'critical view of safety' has been supported and debated in various surveys and reviews [95–97]. However, it is important to recognise that this method is essentially an extension of the '*infundibular view*'.

14.1.2 Technics for exposing and identifying the CD and cystic artery

The first step of laparoscopic cholecystectomy involves a thorough anatomical inspection of the liver and gallbladder. Identifying the location of the gallbladder, its portions, cystic plate, Lund's (Mascagni's) lymph node, anchors, and hepatoduodenal ligament is key. The second step is to locate the Rouvière sulcus and define the non-touch zones posteriorly (G1C and PD potential routes) and anteriorly (AD potential route) by gently flipping Hartmann's pouch in the cephalic, caudal, and lateral directions. Two techniques have been proposed to standardise the exposure of cystic structures and complete laparoscopic cholecystectomy: SS-inner dissection, introduced in 2016 [14], and posterior infundibular dissection, described in 2021 [98, 99].

Both methods use a modified infundibular technique for laparoscopic cholecystectomy and emphasise the importance of exposing the CD, Gn, and their junction. They also encourage critical thinking about the critical view of safety theory, which overemphasises the 'what' (targets) and underestimates the 'how' (actions). Gallbladder surgeons should be familiar with both methods and apply them as needed to expose and identify cystic structures, thereby minimising the risk of bile duct injury during laparoscopic cholecystectomy. In addition, intraoperative techniques such as cholangiography, ultrasonography, and indocyanine green fluorescence imaging can aid in the identification of critical biliary and vascular structures and reduce the likelihood of iatrogenic errors.

14.1.2.1 SS-inner layer exposure technique

This technique involves exposing the SS-inner layer and dissecting the entire gallbladder along this layer. The principal technical steps are as follows:

1. The serosa is incised well above the Rouvière sulcus, at the level of the lower Gb, its posterior wall; close to the juncture of the gallbladder's serosa and liver serosa.

2. SS-outer layer is dissected and ablated, followed by exposure of the SS-innerlayer.

3. SS-inner layer is exposed upwards (upper Gb), downwards (Gn and CD), and backwards (hepatic wall of Gn and Gb) by blunt dissection of the SS-inner and sharp cutting of the serosa and SS-outer, exposing the infundibulum.

4. Steps 1 (behind the sentinel lymph node to start), 2, and 3 are repeated for the anterior wall of the gallbladder.

5. Both the SS-inner layers behind the gallbladder is connected.

6. The infundibulum and CD are isolated, and the hepatocystic triangle is partially exposed.

7. The CD is clipped and transected.

8. The dissection of the Gb is advanced, further exposing the SS-inner and separating it from the SS-outer layer.

9. Division of the thin vessels, which are the branches of the superficial and deep cystic arteries, beneath the SS-inner layer. A shiny membrane (fibrous tissue) may be visible on the SS-inner layer.

In cases of severe acute, chronic, or acute-on-chronic cholecystitis, exposing the SS-inner may not be possible because of the loss of histological architecture and altered tissue texture. In such cases, dissection through the SS-outer layer of the gallbladder is an alternative. Once tissue ablation within the hepatocystic triangle is completed and the cystic artery and duct are identified, dissection between the indurated SS-outer layer and the cystic plate may be performed [14].

14.1.2.2 Posterior infundibular dissection as the primary approach to laparoscopic cholecystectomy

The principal technical steps are as follows:

1. The incision of the peritoneum anterior to the lymphatic node of the lung is at the approximate level of the infundibulum of the gallbladder.

2. The serosal incision is extended laterally toward the CD (around the infundibulum) and posteriorly above the deep branch of the cystic artery toward the Gf.

3. The avascular plane (SS-inner layer) between the deep branch of the cystic artery and the hepatic wall of the gallbladder is exposed by applying medial and cephalad traction to the gallbladder.

4. Complete or nearly complete circumferential dissection of the infundibulum is achieved.

5. Steps 2 and 3 are repeated for dissection of the anterior wall of the gallbladder, above Lund's node, and below the superficial branch of the cystic artery toward the Gf, aided by lateral and superior traction.

6. The CD and cystic artery (within Calot's triangle) are bluntly (usually) dissected to expose the infundibulum and CD.

7. The superficial branch of the cystic artery within the avascular plane beneath the hepatic wall of the gallbladder and posterior to the lymphatic node of Lund is isolated, followed by clipping and division.

8. The CD is clipped and transected.

9. The deep branch of the cystic artery is clipped.

A non-touch zone, implying no skeletonisation of the cystic artery, is referred to as the '*trapezoid of no dissection*' (McElmoyle's shield). It is bordered medially by the common hepatic duct, inferiorly by the lymphatic node of Lund, laterally by the superficial branch of the cystic artery emerging from behind the lymph node, and superiorly by the inferior margin of the liver. It can be expressed as follows: trapezoid of no dissection = hepatocystic triangle – Calot's triangle [98, 99].

14.2 Classification of cholecystectomy based on the completeness of gallbladder resection

According to this criterion, cholecystectomies are classified as total (when the surgical transection plane passes through the CD and the entire Gb is excised) or partial (when part of the gallbladder of any size remains in situ at the end of the surgery).

'*Subtotal cholecystectomy*' is an alternative term for '*partial cholecystectomy*', '*incomplete cholecystectomy*', '*less-than-complete cholecystectomy*', and '*nearly total cholecystectomy*' [100]. Notably, the National Health Service (NHS) in England and the American Medical Association use the term '*partial cholecystectomy*' in their classifications of procedures and interventions [42, 43].

The extent of partial resection varies from approximately 95% removal to wedge resection of the peritoneal wall. Based on technical execution, STCs are classified into four variants: STC-1, STC-2, STC-3, and STC-4 (**Figure 18**) [101].

STC-1 involves the circular excision of a significant portion of the gallbladder. This can be performed in three ways, as shown in **Figure 18**: STC-1A, STC-1B, and STC-1C. STC-2 involves longitudinal excision of the peritoneal wall of the gallbladder with (STC-2A) or without (STC-2B) occlusion and transection of the CD. STC-3 refers to fundectomy and STC-4 refers to wedge resection. The choice of STC modality depends on the surgical pathology, anatomy, and surgeon's experience.

Two broad subtypes of STC, namely open and closed-tract, characterise the procedure of STC [94]. When the lumen of the CD or gallbladder is not obstructed, this subtype is referred to as an open-tract STC. Conversely, when the lumen of the CD or gallbladder remnant is obstructed (by an internal or external suture, metal or plastic clip, or stapler), it is referred to as closed-tract STC. The closed-tract subtype of STC is the primary objective because open-tract STC carries a significant risk of bile leakage from gallbladder remnants. It has been noted that the likelihood of observing bile leakage after open-tract STC exceeds 7-fold [102, 103].

The previously used terms '*fenestrating STC*' and '*reconstituting STC*' [74, 104] do not directly correspond to '*open-tract STC*' and '*closed-tract STC*'. Fenestrating STC is a variant in which the CD is closed at its origin within the gallbladder using a purse-string suture, effectively closing the 'window' (*fenestra in Latin*) to the

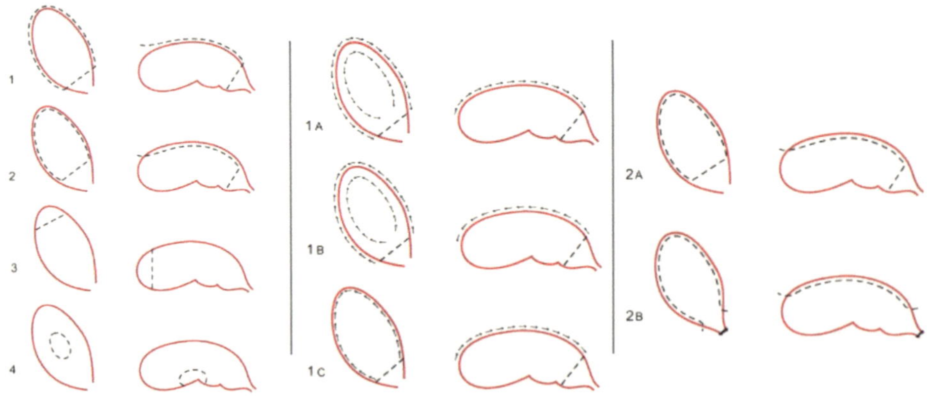

Figure 18.
Four technical variants STC-1, STC-2, STC-3, STC-4, and five subvariants STC-1A, STC-1B, STC-1C, STC-2A, and STC-2B of subtotal cholecystectomy. STC-1A = fundus-downwards technique first, followed by circular transection of the proximal portion of the gallbladder. STC-2B = transection of the proximal portion of the gallbladder first, body-fundus-upwards technique second. STC-1C = partial excision of the peritoneal wall first, the hepatic wall second. STC-2A = resection of the peritoneal wall only. STC-2B = occlusion and transection of the cystic duct, excision of the peritoneal wall, and, if feasible, a portion of the hepatic wall of the gallbladder. The arrowed lines show the direction of detachment of the hepatic wall of the gallbladder from the SS-outer layer or cystic plate. Dotted lines indicate the resection areas [101]. (With approval from the Royal College of Surgeons of England, licenced by the publisher through the Copyright Clearance Centre, Order Licence ID 1580128-1).

rest of the ductal system. This technique transforms open biliary tract surgery into closed-tract surgery [94, 102, 103].

Finally, it is essential to determine when to pause and convert the surgical plan from total cholecystectomy to STC. Despite the numerous indications related to complex pathology, atypical biliary anatomy, human factors, and broader system considerations, a straightforward rule should be followed: conversion to STC (or any other damage-preventing surgery) when further surgical actions may cause injury to the bile duct, major vessels, stomach, intestine or diaphragm. Postoperative morbidity associated with STC is secondary in importance because it is temporary and manageable [85, 102, 105, 106].

14.3 Abandoned cholecystectomy

Cholecystectomy is considered abandoned when a decision is made and acted upon to halt the surgical procedure at any point after the induction of general anaesthesia, regardless of whether a surgical incision was made. It is one of the four bailout procedures in gallbladder surgery [107–109], along with STC (partial), tube cholecystostomy, and cholecystolithotomy [110–112].

Figure 19 illustrates one of the reasons for abandoning laparoscopic cholecystectomy: a chronic pericholecystic inflammatory mass and a non-functional, invisible gallbladder in an asymptomatic patient. Other reasons include suspected malignancy of the gallbladder, liver, or surrounding organs; life-threatening cardiovascular or

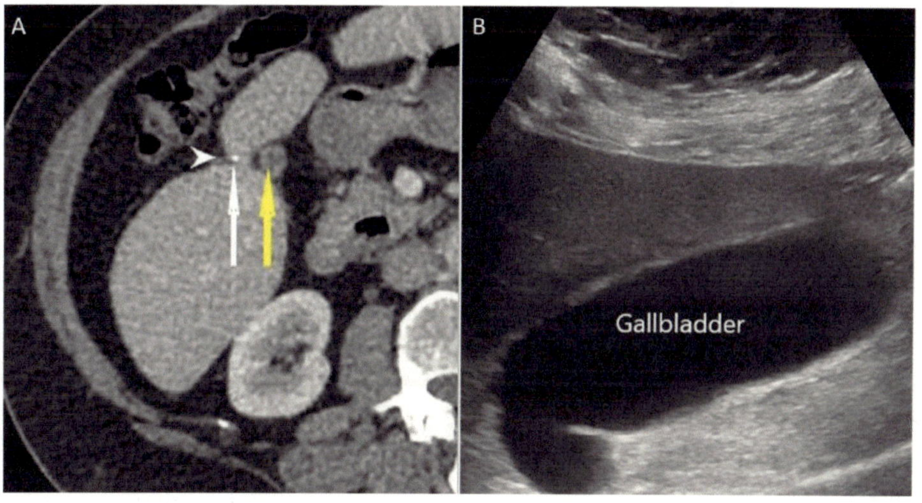

Figure 19.
Images after and before the abandoned cholecystectomy. A: The computed tomography following the abandoned cholecystectomy reveals a severely contracted gallbladder due to chronic fibrotic changes (yellow arrow), with puckering observed between the hemilivers (white arrowhead). The white arrow indicates a small gallstone (or calcified tissue) above the fibrotically contracted gallbladder. B: An ultrasonographic image showing acute calculous cholecystitis, which was conservatively treated 18 months before elective gallbladder surgery. A key clinical point is that the 70-year-old patient was asymptomatic following conservative treatment for acute calculous cholecystitis. This clinical scenario suggests that gallbladder surgery should be cancelled during the preoperative reassessment of the asymptomatic patient on the day of the scheduled procedure (or earlier during a follow-up visit) and further objective investigations should be requested. This also suggests that abandoned cholecystectomy was preventable in this clinical scenario if national and international guidelines and recommendations emphasising the importance of early laparoscopic cholecystectomy for acute calculous cholecystitis had been followed.

respiratory events (such as asystole, severe desaturation, and anaphylactic shock); unforeseen pre-incision incidents related to human factors or complications from gallstone disease; pregnancy as an incidental finding; and lapses in laparoscopic surgical competence.

15. Laparoscopic cholecystectomy for severe cholecystitis and related risks

Severe inflammatory changes in the hepatocytic and Calot's areas, resulting from acute, chronic, or acute-on-chronic inflammation, often complicate the dissection of pericholecystic tissues at every stage of the operation, including the incision of the serosa, ablation of the SS-outer layer, exposure of the SS-inner layer, and identification of the branches or trunk of the cystic artery and duct [113]. Gallbladder surgeons frequently encounter these challenges in emergency cases [51, 80, 114–116].

15.1 Identifying the SS-inner layer as a standard

The third layer of the gallbladder (SS-inner) serves as a proper and safe dissection plane for secure laparoscopic cholecystectomy, even in patients with severe acute or chronic cholecystitis. Accessing this layer *via* the posterior (lateral) peritoneal wall of the gallbladder is considered safe. When surgical access to this part of the gallbladder's peritoneal wall is problematic due to the geometrical features of the gallbladder, the anterior part of the exposed gallbladder's peritoneal wall should be the first surgical target, following an incision through the serosa and the SS-outer layer (see Sections 14.1.2.1 and 14.1.2.2).

Prior to this step, it is crucial to identify non-touch zones to prevent injury to the G1c, Gpost, and Gant pedicles. When laparoscopically inspecting the posterior surface of the cystic pedicle, the first visible pedicle (if observable) should be considered G1c, originating from the caudate process of the liver (**Figure 14**). Gpost is typically situated behind G1c or slightly superior to the Rouvière sulcus ends.

15.2 Exposure of the SS-inner layer and precautionary measures

Following local exposure of the SS-inner layer on either the posterior (preferred) or anterior wall of the gallbladder, continuous blunt dissection should be performed between the SS-inner and SS-outer layers to expose the SS-inner layer. Suction devices are suitable for patients with acute or mild chronic cholecystitis.

Blunt dissection using laparoscopic forceps (e.g., the Maryland dissector), along with careful coagulation diathermy of the exposed tissue bundles, is also effective. However, diathermy should not be used continuously to separate the inner SS layer from the outer SS layers, as this increases the risk of iatrogenic gallbladder perforation, bile and gallstone spillage, loss of gallstones, and a higher likelihood of postoperative infections [117, 118]. Traction with a sharp fundus grasper is another well-known cause of iatrogenic gallbladder fundus injury [119]. Unintentional deviation of the surgical instrument from the SS-inner layer to the fibromuscular layer of the hepatic wall can occur.

Surgeons should exercise caution to prevent gallbladder perforation during laparoscopic cholecystectomy. For example, sharp laparoscopic fundus graspers should be replaced with blunt laparoscopic graspers, particularly in cases involving thin-walled gallbladders.

15.3 Extreme forms of chronic severe cholecystitis and surgery

When well-formed fibrotic tissue or scars replace the subserosal and other layers of the gallbladder, blunt dissection along the boundary between the SS-inner and SS-outer layers or within the hepatocystic area becomes impossible. This condition is often observed in small, shrunken gallbladders and represents a manifestation of chronic cholecystitis. The adjacent liver parenchyma (pucker sign) [120], as well as the intrahepatic, subvesical (Luschka), cystic, and extrahepatic bile ducts and vessels, may also be involved in a severe chronic pericholecystic inflammatory process, resulting in an inflammatory mass.

In such hazardous scenarios, the decision to convert gallbladder surgery to STC or other bailout-type surgical procedures should be made swiftly. Ineffective attempts to obtain a critical view of safety and anatomically excise the hepatic wall of the gallbladder may lead to clinically significant bleeding from the surrounding veins and arteries or injury to the bile duct. Ideally, shared decision-making should be the standard practice in non-standard situations. Damage control surgical procedures are common in England and the United States [100, 121–125].

15.4 Division of the subserosal layer in instances of suppurative, necrotic, gangrenous, or emphysematous cholecystitis

Gallbladder tissue separation depends on the features of acute cholecystitis (**Figure 20**). For instance, employing an irrigation-suction device (hydrodissection) within the infected SS-outer layer or at the junction of the outer SS layer and the cystic plate is often a practical choice, yielding optimal clinical outcomes. It is also important to note that small liver abscesses suspected preoperatively are often pus collections within the outer SS layer. In such instances, the outer SS layer within the pus collection zone appears as an amorphous, grey, soft mass. Hydrodissection and blunt dissection are effective methods for tissue separation during emergency laparoscopic cholecystectomy. Although infection-induced injury to the Luschka duct is a theoretical concern, this scenario remains unlikely.

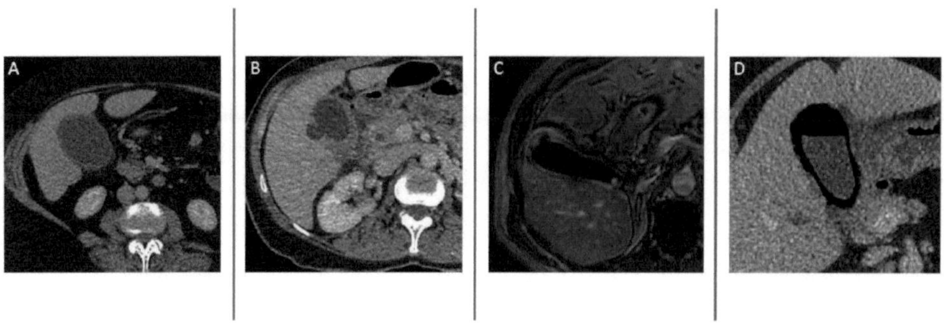

Figure 20.
*Acute calculous cholecystitis confirmed using computed tomography (CT) or magnetic resonance imaging (MRI). A: The diagnosis of acute cholecystitis is based on a CT scan. Emergency laparoscopic surgery revealed suppurative calculous cholecystitis (empyema of the gallbladder); subtotal cholecystectomy (95% volume STC-1A, open-tract) was performed (***Figure 18***) [94, 101–103]. B: Acute perforated calculous cholecystitis with perforation in segment 5. A laparoscopic subtotal cholecystectomy (STC-2B) was performed, and the abscess was found within the outer subserosal layer. C: MRI revealed perforation and fluid collection (likely infected) within the outer, subserosal layer. D: Emphysematous and gangrenous perforated cholecystitis, with extensive pericholecystic inflammatory changes reported. A laparoscopic total cholecystectomy was performed.*

15.5 The pitfalls of fundus-down cholecystectomy

First, when the fundus-down approach is required for total conventional or STC, the SS-inner layer, which is thin at the anterior aspect of the Gf, should be exposed with utmost caution.

Second, detaching the SS-outer layer of the hepatic wall of the gallbladder from the cystic plate toward its neck may risk injuring the right-sided Glissonian pedicles, right hepatic duct, or even the common hepatic duct [126–129]. This complication typically occurs in an unfavourable local surgical environment, particularly when oozing from the tissues of the gallbladder hepatic wall or damaged liver parenchyma persists.

When feasible, tunnelling the SS-outer layer at the level of the lower Gb before starting fundus-down dissection facilitates the procedure. This technique creates a surgical marker indicating that further dissection should be slowed or halted. Alternative strategies include opening the gallbladder cavity to better control the dissection of the hepatic wall. STC, classified as STC-1C (removal of the peritoneal wall first, followed by removal of the hepatic wall) [101], is the third option for preventing the undesirable side effects of fundus-down cholecystectomy.

Third, understanding sectional liver anatomy and being aware of the non-touch zones, Gant and Gpost, are crucial when performing surgery for benign gallbladder disease or precancerous conditions, such as a 'porcelain' gallbladder. Even within the context of oncological hepatobiliary surgery, performing a five-layer (cystic plate) or six-layer (full-thickness) cholecystectomy for suspected malignant disease requires a meticulous technique.

15.6 Statistical insights into risks in laparoscopic cholecystectomy

Several statistical figures warrant further investigations. The United Kingdom's CholeS snapshot audit revealed that 9% of laparoscopic cholecystectomies performed in approximately 9000 patients were challenging. The injury rate among patients with intraoperative cholecystectomy difficulty grade 4/5 was 1.7%, which is more than 56 times greater than the injury rate for grade 1 difficulty, 9–10 times greater than that for grades 2 or 3, and almost 7 times greater than the overall bile duct injury rate of 0.25% [130]. Furthermore, two systematic reviews on left-sided gallbladders highlighted unacceptably high iatrogenic bile duct injury rates of 4.4 and 7.3%, respectively [62].

This indirectly indicates that most bile duct injuries occur during dissection of the hepatocystic area, which is performed to comply with the key requirement of the critical window of safety theory: exposing only two structures, the cystic artery and the duct. This is performed after ablative dissection within the hepatocystic triangle and proximal third of the hepatic wall.

Surgeons operating on adjacent organs must have a fundamental understanding of biliary anatomy. A rare but catastrophic scenario involves a right portal pedicle injury during right nephrectomy, which may require immediate vascular intervention and urgent, life-saving right hepatectomy.

16. Concluding remarks

1. Over the past 50 years, significant advancements have been made in understanding the systematic and topographical anatomies of the gallbladder and bile ducts.

2. Although Latin dominated medical sciences in Europe for nearly 20 centuries, it was swiftly replaced by the national languages within a few decades.

3. Eponyms for liver and biliary anatomy remain deeply embedded in anatomical and surgical terminology, while new theories of biliary anatomy continue to evolve alongside advancements in liver surgery, enhancing both clinical and anatomical accuracy.

4. Clarifying the relationship between the hepatic plate, including the cystic plate, and Laënnec's capsule has provided a theoretical foundation for novel hepatobiliary surgical approaches and injury prevention during cholecystectomy.

5. The classification of subsegmental, segmental, and sectional (sectorial) portal pedicles and bile ducts follows a division-based hierarchy, making the term 'aberrant' inappropriate due to its lack of precision in describing biliary anatomy or surgical outcomes.

6. The contemporary description of the gallbladder's cross-sectional structure—a five-layer peritoneal wall and a six-layer hepatic wall—has practical implications in both non-oncological and oncological contexts, with the six-layer hepatic wall theory particularly valuable in oncology.

7. The stratification of the SS layer of the gallbladder into two distinct layers, the SS-inner and SS-outer, has redefined the surgical approach to traditional cholecystectomy.

8. Standardising conventional laparoscopic cholecystectomy by exposing the SS-inner layer and revealing key structures of the cystic pedicle, including the cystic artery or its branches and the cystic duct, enhanced anatomical precision and surgical safety.

9. Both the SS-inner layer and posterior infundibular techniques for exposing cystic structures are conceptually interdependent with a critical view of safety theory.

10. Acute and chronic cholecystitis can significantly alter the cross-sectional structures of the gallbladder and bile ducts, necessitating flexible surgical strategies to preserve bile duct integrity.

11. In extraordinary circumstances such as severe biliary disease, unusual surgical anatomy, or human factors, alternative procedures to the conventional three-layer cholecystectomy—including subtotal cholecystectomy, cholecystolithotomy, tube cholecystostomy, and abandoned cholecystectomy—must be considered.

12. Ultimately, precise documentation of preoperative, intraoperative, and postoperative findings is essential, necessitating continuous study of the systematic, topographical, and surgical anatomy of the gallbladder and bile ducts as a fundamental component of precision surgery.

Author details

Raimundas Lunevicius
Department of Emergency General Surgery, Aintree University Hospital, NHS University Hospitals of Liverpool Group, UK

*Address all correspondence to: raimundas.lunevicius@liverpoolft.nhs.uk

References

[1] Mahadevan V. Anatomy of the gallbladder and bile ducts. Surgery (Oxford). 2020;**38**:432-436. DOI: 10.1016/j.mpsur.2014.10.003

[2] Williams PL, Warwick R, editors. The biliary ducts and gall bladder. In: Gray's Anatomy. 36th ed. Churchill Livingstone, Edinburgh, London, Melbourne, New York: Medical Division of Longman Group Limited; 1980. pp. 1382-1385

[3] Healey JE Jr, Schroy PC. Anatomy of the biliary ducts within the human liver; analysis of the prevailing pattern of branchings and the major variations of the biliary ducts. AMA Archives of Surgery. 1953;**66**:599-616. DOI: 10.1001/archsurg.1953.01260030616008

[4] Couinaud C. Surgical Anatomy of the Liver Revisited. Paris: C. Couinaud; 1989

[5] Wise PE, Holzman MD. Surgical anatomy of the gallbladder, liver, and biliary tree. In: MacFadyen BV et al., editors. Laparoscopic Surgery of the Abdomen. New York: Springer; 2004. pp. 73-86

[6] Crawford JM. Liver and biliary tract. In: Kumar V, Abbas AK, Fausto N, editors. Robbins and Cotran Pathologic Basis of Disease. 7th ed. Philadelphia: Saunders Elsevier; 2005. pp. 877-937

[7] Ahmed S, Tuttle-Newhall JE. Liver anatomy and anatomic variants. In: Blazer DG III, Kuo PC, Pappas T, Clary BM, editors. Contemporary Surgical Management of Liver, Biliary Tract, and Pancreatic Disease. World Scientific Co Pte, Ltd; 2013. pp. 3-19. Available from: https://www.worldscientific.com/doi/abs/10.1142/9789814293068_0001

[8] Gill RM, Theise ND. Rappaport, Glisson, Hering, and mall-champions of liver microanatomy: Microscopic and ultramicroscopic anatomy of the liver into the modern age. Clinical Liver Disease (Hoboken). 2021;**18**(Suppl. 1):76-92. DOI: 10.1002/cld.1145

[9] van Gulik TM. Liver anatomy by Francis Glisson. Hepatobiliary Surgery and Nutrition. 2022;**11**:502-503. DOI: 10.21037/hbsn-2022-17

[10] Strasberg SM, Belghiti J, Clavien PA, et al. The Brisbane 2000 terminology of liver anatomy and resections. HPB. 2000;**2**:333-339

[11] Strasberg SM. Nomenclature of hepatic anatomy and resections: A review of the Brisbane 2000 system. Journal of Hepato-Biliary-Pancreatic Surgery. 2005;**12**:351-355. DOI: 10.1007/s00534-005-0999-7

[12] Strasberg SM, Phillips C. Use and dissemination of the Brisbane 2000 nomenclature of liver anatomy and resections. Annals of Surgery. 2013;**257**:377-382. DOI: 10.1097/SLA.0b013e31825a01f6

[13] Honda G, Iwanaga T, Kurata M, et al. The critical view of safety in laparoscopic cholecystectomy is optimized by exposing the inner layer of the subserosal layer. Journal of Hepato-Biliary-Pancreatic Surgery. 2009;**16**:445-449. DOI: 10.1007/s00534-009-0060-3

[14] Honda G, Hasegawa H, Umezawa A. Universal safe procedure of laparoscopic cholecystectomy standardized by exposing the inner layer of the subserosal layer (with video). Journal of Hepato-Biliary-Pancreatic Sciences. 2016;**23**:E14-E19. DOI: 10.1002/jhbp.382

[15] Roy PG, Soonawalla ZF, Grant HW. Medicolegal costs of bile duct injuries incurred during laparoscopic cholecystectomy. HPB: The Official Journal of the International Hepato Pancreato Biliary Association. 2009;**11**:130-134. DOI: 10.1111/j.1477-2574.2008.00023.x

[16] Landman MP, Feurer ID, Moore DE, et al. The long-term effect of bile duct injuries on health-related quality of life: A meta-analysis. HPB: The Official Journal of the International Hepato Pancreato Biliary Association. 2013;**15**:252-259. DOI: 10.1111/j.1477-2574.2012.00586.x

[17] Hariharan D, Psaltis E, Scholefield JH, Lobo DN. Quality of life and medico-legal implications following iatrogenic bile duct injuries. World Journal of Surgery. 2017;**41**:90-99. DOI: 10.1007/s00268-016-3677-9

[18] Cirocchi R, Panata L, Griffiths EA, et al. Injuries during laparoscopic cholecystectomy: A scoping review of the claims and civil action judgements. Journal of Clinical Medicine. 2021;**10**:5238. DOI: 10.3390/jcm10225238

[19] Reinsoo A, Kirsimägi Ü, Kibuspuu L, et al. Bile duct injuries during laparoscopic cholecystectomies: An 11-year population-based study. European Journal of Trauma and Emergency Surgery. 2023;**49**:2269-2276. DOI: 10.1007/s00068-022-02190-9

[20] Pang YY. The Brisbane 2000 terminology of liver anatomy and resections. HPB: The Official Journal of the International Hepato Pancreato Biliary Association. 2002;**4**:99-100. DOI: 10.1080/136518202760378489

[21] Baethge C, Goldbeck-Wood S, Mertens S. SANRA-a scale for the quality assessment of narrative review articles. Research Integration and Peer Review. 2019;**4**:5. DOI: 10.1186/s41073-019-0064-8

[22] Royal College of Obstetricians and Gynaecologists. Presenting information on risk. In: Clinical Governance Advice No. 7. London: RCOG; 2009. Available from: https://www.rcog.org.uk/globalassets/documents/guidelines/clinical-governance-advice/cga7-15072010.pdf

[23] Spirou Y, Petrou A, Christoforides C, Felekouras E. History of biliary surgery. World Journal of Surgery. 2013;**37**:1006-1012. DOI: 10.1007/s00268-013-1960-6. Erratum in: World Journal of Surgery. 2013;37:1748. Yannos, Spirou [corrected to Spirou, Yannos]; Athanasios, Petrou [corrected to Petrou, Athanasios]; Christos, Christoforides [corrected to Christoforides, Christos]; Evangelos, Felekouras [corrected to Felekouras, Evangelos]

[24] Wood M. Presidential address: Eponyms in biliary tract surgery. American Journal of Surgery. 1979;**138**:746-754. DOI: 10.1016/0002-9610(79)90290-3

[25] Hayashi S, Murakami G, Ohtsuka A, et al. Connective tissue configuration in the human liver hilar region with special reference to the liver capsule and vascular sheath. Journal of Hepato-Biliary-Pancreatic Surgery. 2008;**15**:640-647. DOI: 10.1007/s00534-008-1336-8

[26] Sugioka A, Kato Y, Tanahashi Y. Systematic extrahepatic Glissonean pedicle isolation for anatomical liver resection based on Laennec's capsule: Proposal of a novel comprehensive surgical anatomy of the liver. Journal of Hepato-Biliary-Pancreatic Sciences. 2017;**24**:17-23. DOI: 10.1002/jhbp.410

[27] Davies F, Harding HE. The pouch of Hartmann. The Lancet.

1942;**239**:193-195. DOI: 10.1016/S0140-6736(00)79463-3

[28] Walsh TH, Akoglu T, Chandra M, Osung O. The muscle content of the mammalian cystic duct – Does an anatomical sphincter exist? Annals of the Royal College of Surgeons of England. 1985;**67**:53

[29] Housset C, Chrétien Y, Debray D, Chignard N. Functions of the gallbladder. Comprehensive Physiology. 2016;**6**:1549-1577. DOI: 10.1002/cphy.c150050

[30] Pina LN, Samoilovich F, Urrutia S, et al. Surgical considerations of the cystic duct and heister valves. The Surgery Journal (NY). 2015;**1**:e23-e27. DOI: 10.1055/s-0035-1567879

[31] Hirota M, Takada T, Kawarada Y, et al. Diagnostic criteria and severity assessment of acute cholecystitis: Tokyo guidelines. Journal of Hepato-Biliary-Pancreatic Surgery. 2007;**14**:78-82. DOI: 10.1007/s00534-006-1159-4

[32] Yokoe M, Hata J, Takada T, et al. Tokyo guidelines 2018: Diagnostic criteria and severity grading of acute cholecystitis (with videos). Journal of Hepato-Biliary-Pancreatic Sciences. 2018;**25**:41-54. DOI: 10.1002/jhbp.515

[33] Mayumi T, Okamoto K, Takada T, et al. Tokyo guidelines 2018: Management bundles for acute cholangitis and cholecystitis. Journal of Hepato-Biliary-Pancreatic Sciences. 2018;**25**:96-100. DOI: 10.1002/jhbp.519

[34] Hugh TB, Kelly MD, Mekisic A. Rouvière's sulcus: A useful landmark in laparoscopic cholecystectomy. British Journal of Surgery. 1997;**84**:1253-1254. DOI: 10.1046/j.1365-2168.1997.02769.x

[35] Singh M, Prasad N. The anatomy of Rouviere's sulcus as seen during laparoscopic cholecystectomy: A proposed classification. Journal of Minimal Access Surgery. 2017;**13**:89-95. DOI: 10.4103/0972-9941.201731

[36] Aoki S, Mizuma M, Hayashi H, et al. Surgical anatomy of the right hepatic artery in Rouviere's sulcus evaluated by preoperative multidetector-row CT images. BMC Surgery. 2016;**16**:40. DOI: 10.1186/s12893-016-0155-0

[37] Abdalla S, Pierre S, Ellis H. Calot's triangle. Clinical Anatomy. 2013;**26**:493-501. DOI: 10.1002/ca.22170

[38] Sakamoto Y, Kokudo N, Kawaguchi Y, Akita K. Clinical anatomy of the liver: Review of the 19th Meeting of the Japanese Research Society of Clinical Anatomy. Liver Cancer. 2017;**6**:146-160. DOI: 10.1159/000449490

[39] Banerjee A, Hariharan D. History of liver surgery. Clinical Liver Disease (Hoboken). 2024;**23**:e0237. DOI: 10.1097/CLD.0000000000000237

[40] Ko K, Kamiya J, Nagino M, et al. A study of the subvesical bile duct (duct of Luschka) in resected liver specimens. World Journal of Surgery. 2006;**30**:1316-1320. DOI: 10.1007/s00268-005-0469-z

[41] Belarry SS, Walters A, Gielecki J, et al. Winslow (1669-1760). Clinical Anatomy. 2012;**25**:545-547. DOI: 10.1002/ca.22033

[42] NHS Digital. Classifications browser OPCS – 4.9. Available from https://classbrowser.nhs.uk/#/book/OPCS-4.9 [Accessed: March 25, 2025]

[43] Surgery CPT® Code Range 10004-69990. American Medical Association. Available from: https://www.aapc.com/codes/cpt-codes-range/10004-69990/ [Accessed: March 25, 2025]

[44] Pasternak A, Gajda M, Gil K, et al. Evidence of interstitial Cajal-like cells in human gallbladder. Folia Histochemica et Cytobiologica. 2012;**50**:581-585. DOI: 10.5603/19673

[45] Classification of Biliary Tract Carcinoma. Japanese Society of Biliary Surgery (JSBS). 2nd English ed. Tokyo: Kanehara & Co.; 2004

[46] Miyazaki M, Ohtsuka M, Miyakawa S, et al. Classification of biliary tract cancers established by the Japanese Society of Hepato-Biliary-Pancreatic Surgery: 3rd English edition. Journal of Hepato-Biliary-Pancreatic Sciences. 2015;**22**:181-196. DOI: 10.1002/jhbp.211

[47] Honda G, Iwanaga T, Kurata M. Dissection of the gallbladder from the liver bed during laparoscopic cholecystectomy for acute or subacute cholecystitis. Journal of Hepato-Biliary-Pancreatic Surgery. 2008;**15**:293-296. DOI: 10.1007/s00534-007-1260-3

[48] Honda G, Iwasaki K, Matsumura H, et al. Through which layer, between the gallbladder and the liver, does the deep branch of the cystic artery run? Asian Journal of Endoscopic Surgery. 2010;**3**:192-195. DOI: 10.1111/j.1758-5910.2010.00056.x

[49] Sugioka A et al. Cystic plate cholecystectomy, Laennec's capsule and hepatic plate system. In: Yamamoto M, Conrad C, editors. 解剖を理解し手術を究める 肝胆膵外科手術 Japanese Mastery in Hepato-Pancreato-Biliary Surgery. Tokyo: Gakken Medical Shujunsha Co., Ltd; 2021. pp. 2-11. ISBN-13 9784780904284

[50] Endo I. Hepatic plate and portal vascular dissection. In: Yamamoto M, Conrad C, editors. 解剖を理解し手術を究める 肝胆膵外科手術 Japanese Mastery in Hepato-Pancreato-Biliary Surgery. Tokyo: Gakken Medical Shujunsha Co., Ltd; 2021. pp. 12-17. ISBN-13 9784780904284

[51] Iwashita Y, Ohyama T, Honda G, et al. What are the appropriate indicators of surgical difficulty during laparoscopic cholecystectomy? Results from a Japan-Korea-Taiwan multinational survey. Journal of Hepato-Biliary-Pancreatic Sciences. 2016;**23**:533-547. DOI: 10.1002/jhbp.375

[52] Huang TL, Cheng YF, Chen CL, et al. Variants of the bile ducts: Clinical application in the potential donor of living-related hepatic transplantation. Transplantation Proceedings. 1996;**28**:1669-1670

[53] Ohkubo M, Nagino M, Kamiya J, et al. Surgical anatomy of the bile ducts at the hepatic hilum as applied to living donor liver transplantation. Annals of Surgery. 2004;**239**:82-86. DOI: 10.1097/01.sla.0000102934.93029.89

[54] Olmedo NB, Dos Santos JS, Junior JE. The frequency of anatomical variants of the bile ducts: A review based on a single classification as support for cholangiographic examinations. Cureus. 2024;**16**:e58905. DOI: 10.7759/cureus.58905

[55] Meedeniya AC, Schloithe AC, Toouli J, Saccone GT. Characterization of the intrinsic and extrinsic innervation of the gall bladder epithelium in the Australian brush-tailed possum (Trichosurus vulpecula). Neurogastroenterology & Motility. 2003;**15**:383-392. DOI: 10.1046/j.1365-2982.2003.00417.x

[56] Ding F, Hu Q, Wang Y, et al. Smooth muscle cells, interstitial cells and neurons in the gallbladder (GB): Functional

syncytium of electrical rhythmicity and GB motility (review). International Journal of Molecular Medicine. 2023;**51**:33. DOI: 10.3892/ijmm.2023.5236

[57] Deutschmann K, Reich M, Klindt C, et al. Bile acid receptors in the biliary tree: TGR5 in physiology and disease. Biochimica et Biophysica Acta (BBA) - Molecular Basis of Disease. 2018;**1864**(4 Pt. B):1319-1325. DOI: 10.1016/j.bbadis.2017.08.021

[58] Kim YC, Seok S, Zhang Y, et al. Intestinal FGF15/19 physiologically repress hepatic lipogenesis in the late fed-state by activating SHP and DNMT3A. Nature Communications. 2020;**11**:5969. DOI: 10.1038/s41467-020-19803-9

[59] Bates JA, Dinnan K, Sharp V. Biliary hyperkinesia, a new diagnosis or misunderstood pathophysiology of dyskinesia: A case report. International Journal of Surgical Case Reports. 2019;**55**:80-83. DOI: 10.1016/j.ijscr.2019.01.011

[60] Cotton PB, Elta GH, Carter CR, et al. Gallbladder and sphincter of Oddi disorders. Gastroenterology. 2016;**150**:1420-1429. S0016-5085(16)00224-9. DOI: 10.1053/j.gastro.2016.02.033

[61] van Kamp MJ, Bouman DE, Steenvoorde P, Klaase JM. A phrygian cap. Case Reports in Gastroenterology. 2013;7:347-351. DOI: 10.1159/000354789

[62] Lunevicius R, Chawdhery MZ, Jones J. Subtotal cholecystectomy as an approach to preventing injury in the left-sided gallbladder in the emergency surgery setting: A case study. Journal of Clinical and Translational Research. 2024;**10**:9-17. DOI: 10.36922/jctr.00128

[63] Alharthi S, Bernon M, Krige JE. Beware the left-sided gallbladder. South African Journal of Surgery. 2012;**50**:88-89. DOI: 10.7196/sajs.1301

[64] Arora GS, Kalra S. Ectopic liver tissue encountered incidentally during a laparoscopic cholecystectomy: A case report. Cureus. 2023;**15**:e42220. DOI: 10.7759/cureus.42220

[65] Terkawi RS, Qutob D, Hendaus MA. Understanding multiseptated gallbladder: A systematic analysis with a case report. Journal of Gastroenterology and Hepatology Open. 2021;**5**:988-996. DOI: 10.1002/jgh3.12621

[66] Baz C, Nudotor R, Buseey I, Stitely K. Rare finding of ectopic pancreas in a cholecystectomy specimen: Case report and literature review. Journal of Surgical Case Reports. 2024;**2024**(10):rjae659. DOI: 10.1093/jscr/rjae659

[67] Carbajo MA, Martín del Omo JC, Blanco JI, et al. Congenital malformations of the gallbladder and cystic duct diagnosed by laparoscopy: High surgical risk. Journal of the Society of Laparoscopic & Robotic Surgeons. 1999;**3**:319-321

[68] Piltcher-da-Silva R, Sasaki VL, Felisberto DEG, et al. Gallbladder agenesis a rare and underdiagnosed congenital anomaly: A case report and literature review. Journal of Surgical Case Reports. 2022;**2022**(11):1-4. DOI: 10.1093/jscr/rjac505

[69] Raparia K, Zhai QJ, Schwartz MR, et al. Muscularis mucosae versus muscularis propria in gallbladder, cystic duct, and common bile duct: Smoothelin and desmin immunohistochemical study. Annals of Diagnostic Pathology. 2010;**14**:408-412. DOI: 10.1016/j.anndiagpath.2010.05.013

[70] Tryantafyllou G, Belimezakis N, Lyros O, et al. Surgical anatomy of the

cystic artery: A systematic review with meta-analysis. Annals of Anatomy. 2025;**257**:152343. DOI: 10.1016/j.aanat.2024.152343

[71] Kim SH, Park S, Choi J. A cystic artery arising from the middle hepatic artery detected during laparoscopic cholecystectomy: A case report. Journal of Surgical Case Reports. 2022;**2022**(1):rjab088. DOI: 10.1093/jscr/rjab088

[72] Perdikakis M, Liapi A, Kiriakopoulos A, et al. Anatomical variations of the cystic artery and laparoscopic cholecystectomy: A persisting surgical challenge. Cureus. 2024;**16**:e67948. DOI: 10.7759/cureus.67948

[73] Tiang KW, Peng JX, Wysocki AP. Cystic artery lymph node: Is it a fixed important landmark during cholecystectomy. Liver and Pancreatic Sciences. 2017;**2**:1-2. DOI: 10.15761/LPS.1000114

[74] Strasberg SM. A three-step conceptual roadmap for avoiding bile duct injury in laparoscopic cholecystectomy: An invited perspective review. Journal of Hepato-Biliary-Pancreatic Sciences. 2019;**26**:123-127. DOI: 10.1002/jhbp.616

[75] Koo JGA, Tham HY, Toh EQ, et al. Mirizzi syndrome-the past, present, and future. Medicina (Kaunas, Lithuania). 2023;**60**:12. DOI: 10.3390/medicina60010012

[76] Tokumitsu Y, Shindo Y, Matsui H, et al. Laparoscopic total biopsy for suspected gallbladder cancer: A case series. Health Science Report. 2020;**3**:e156. DOI: 10.1002/hsr2.156

[77] Tokumitsu Y, Tamesa T, Shindo Y, et al. Application and utility of surgical techniques for cystic plate isolation in liver surgery. Annals of Gastroenterological Surgery. 2022;**6**:726-732. DOI: 10.1002/ags3.12568

[78] Takasaki K. Glissonean pedicle transection method for hepatic resection: A new concept of liver segmentation. Journal of Hepato-Biliary-Pancreatic Surgery. 1998;**5**:286-291. DOI: 10.1007/s005340050047

[79] Sugioka A, Kato Y, Tanahashi Y, et al. Standardization of anatomic liver resection based on Laennec's capsule. Surgery, Gastroenterology and Oncology. 2020;**25**:57. DOI: 10.21614/sgo-25-2-57

[80] Ome Y et al. Cholecystectomy for acute cholecystitis. In: Yamamoto M, Conrad C, editors. 解剖を理解し手術を究める 肝胆膵外科手術 Japanese Mastery in Hepato-Pancreato-Biliary Surgery. Tokyo: Gakken Medical Shujunsha Co., Ltd; 2021. pp. 27-34. ISBN-13 9784780904284

[81] Ciria R, Ayllón MD, Briceño J. Liver gates to access everywhere in the liver: How can we learn? Digestive Medicine Research. 2023;**6**:1-7. DOI: 10.21037/dmr-22-66

[82] Strasberg SM, Hertl M, Soper NJ. An analysis of the problem of biliary injury during laparoscopic cholecystectomy. Journal of the American College of Surgeons. 1995;**180**:101-125

[83] Bektas H, Schrem H, Winny M, Klempnauer J. Surgical treatment and outcome of iatrogenic bile duct lesions after cholecystectomy and the impact of different clinical classification systems. Journal of British Surgery. 2007;**94**:1119-1127. DOI: 10.1002/bjs.5752

[84] Castaing D. Surgical anatomy of the biliary tract. HPB: The Official Journal of the International Hepato Pancreato

Biliary Association. 2008;**10**:72-76. DOI: 10.1080/13651820801992518

[85] Lunevicius R, Haagsma JA. Supplementary material to 'subtotal cholecystectomy: Results of a single-Centre, registry-based retrospective cohort study of 180 adults in 2011-2018'. Mendeley Data. 2002. V1. DOI: 10.17632/khv3b7b6wf.1. Available from: https://data.mendeley.com/datasets/khv3b7b6wf/1

[86] Avisse C, Flament JB, Delattre JF. Ampulla of Vater. Anatomic, embryologic, and surgical aspects. Surgical Clinics of North America. 2000;**80**:201-212. DOI: 10.1016/s0039-6109(05)70402-3

[87] Persaud T, Dawod E, Shah S, et al. A tale of two ampullas: A rare anatomic anomaly captured on video during endoscopic retrograde cholangiopancreatography. Endoscopy. 2023;**55**(S01):E78-E79. DOI: 10.1055/a-1930-6202

[88] Bains L, Pradhan U. Safety landmarks in laparoscopic cholecystectomy [Internet]. In: Gallstone Disease - Newer Insights and Current Trends. London, UK: IntechOpen; 2024. DOI: 10.5772/intechopen.113223. Available from: Safety Landmarks in Laparoscopic Cholecystectomy | IntechOpen

[89] Ozden I, Kamiya J, Nagino M, et al. Clinicoanatomical study on the infraportal bile ducts of segment 3. World Journal of Surgery. 2002;**26**:1441-1445. DOI: 10.1007/s00268-002-6544-9

[90] Kamiya J, Nagino M, Uesaka K, et al. Clinicoanatomical studies on the dorsal subsegmental bile duct of the right anterior superior segment of the human liver. Langenbeck's Archives of Surgery. 2003;**388**:107-111. DOI: 10.1007/s00423-003-0373-7

[91] Wang SD, Wang L, Xiao H, et al. Novel techniques of liver segmental and subsegmental pedicle anatomy from segment 1 to segment 8. World Journal of Gastrointestinal Surgery. 2024;**16**:3806-3817. DOI: 10.4240/wjgs.v16.i12.3806

[92] Wakabayashi G, Cherqui D, Geller DA, et al. The Tokyo 2020 terminology of liver anatomy and resections: Updates of the Brisbane 2000 system. Journal of Hepato-Biliary-Pancreatic Sciences. 2022;**29**:6-15. DOI: 10.1002/jhbp.1091

[93] National Confidential Enquiry into Patient Outcome and Death. The NCEPOD classification of interventions. Available from: https://www.ncepod.org.uk/classification.html [Accessed: January 23, 2025]

[94] Lunevicius R. Review of the literature on partial resections of the gallbladder, 1898-2022: The outline of the conception of subtotal cholecystectomy and a suggestion to use the terms 'subtotal open-tract cholecystectomy' and 'subtotal closed-tract cholecystectomy'. Journal of Clinical Medicine. 2023;**12**:1230. DOI: 10.3390/jcm12031230

[95] Brunt LM, Deziel DJ, Telem DA, et al. Safe cholecystectomy multi-society practice guideline and state of the art consensus conference on prevention of bile duct injury during cholecystectomy. Annals of Surgery. 2020;**272**:3-23. DOI: 10.1097/SLA.0000000000003791

[96] Sgaramella LI, Gurrado A, Pasculli A, et al. The critical view of safety during laparoscopic cholecystectomy: Strasberg yes or No? An Italian multicentre study. Surgical Endoscopy. 2021;**35**:3698-3708. DOI: 10.1007/s00464-020-07852-6

[97] Montalvo-Javé EE, Contreras-Flores EH, Ayala-Moreno EA,

Mercado MA. Strasberg's critical view: Strategy for a safe laparoscopic cholecystectomy. Euroasian Journal of Hepato-gastroenterology. 2022;**12**:40-44. DOI: 10.5005/jp-journals-10018-1353

[98] Hoang CM, Ferzli G. Being critical of the critical view of safety: Alternate approach in the armamentarium for laparoscopic cholecystectomy. Annals of Laparoscopic and Endoscopic Surgery. 2024;**9**:21. DOI: 10.21037/ales-23-62

[99] Iskandar M, Fingerhut A, Ferzli G. Posterior infundibular dissection: Safety first in laparoscopic cholecystectomy. Surgical Endoscopy. 2021;**35**:3175-3183. DOI: 10.1007/s00464-020-08281-1

[100] Lunevicius R. Insights from global, national, and local studies of benign biliary disease for 2023. In: Lunevicius R, editor. Gallstone Disease—Newer Insights and Current Trends. London, UK: IntechOpen; 2024. DOI: 10.5772/intechopen.114994. Available from: https://www.intechopen.com/chapters/89410

[101] Lunevicius R. Laparoscopic subtotal cholecystectomy: A classification, which encompasses the variants, technical modalities, and extent of resection of the gallbladder. Annals of Royal College of Surgeons of England. 2020;**102**:315-317. DOI: 10.1308/rcsann.2020.0007

[102] Lunevicius R, Nzenwa IC. Multiple logistic regression model to predict bile leak associated with subtotal cholecystectomy. Surgical Endoscopy. 2023;**37**:5405-5413. DOI: 10.1007/s00464-023-10049-2

[103] Lunevicius R, Nzenwa IC. Supplemental data content to 'data from 81 cases of subtotal cholecystectomy used to generate a multiple logistic regression model to predict postoperative bile leak'. Mendeley Data. 2023. V2. DOI: 10.17632/sfvdkmxvbp.2. Available from: https://data.mendeley.com/datasets/sfvdkmxvbp/2

[104] Strasberg SM, Pucci MJ, Brunt LM, Deziel DJ. Subtotal cholecystectomy-"Fenestrating" vs "reconstituting" subtypes and the prevention of bile duct injury: Definition of the optimal procedure in difficult operative conditions. Journal of the American College of Surgeons. 2016;**222**:89-96. DOI: 10.1016/j.jamcollsurg.2015.09.019

[105] Lunevicius R, Haagsma JA. Subtotal cholecystectomy: Results of a single-center, registry-based retrospective cohort study of 180 adults in 2011-2018. Journal of Laparoendoscopic & Advanced Surgical Techniques. Part A. 2021;**31**:1019-1033. DOI: 10.1089/lap.2020.0713

[106] Nzenwa IC, Mesri M, Lunevicius R. Risks associated with subtotal cholecystectomy and the factors influencing them: A systematic review and meta-analysis of 85 studies published between 1985 and 2020. Surgery. 2021;**170**:1014-1023. DOI: 10.1016/j.surg.2021.03.036

[107] Panni UY, Williams GA, Hammill CW, et al. Cause and outcome of aborting a difficult laparoscopic cholecystectomy due to severe inflammation: A study of operative notes. Surgical Endoscopy. 2022;**36**:7288-7294. DOI: 10.1007/s00464-022-09110-3

[108] Julius B, Bolger J, O'Brien L, et al. Abandoned laparoscopic cholecystectomy: A safe strategy for managing the difficult gallbladder. Mesentery and Peritoneum. 2020;**4**:AB019. DOI: 10.21037/map.2020.AB019

[109] Jawad Z, Draz A, Pencavel T, Jiao L. Abandonment and referral of the

difficult laparoscopic cholecystectomy: An excellent alternative management strategy. HPB. 2016;**18**(S1):e385-e601. Available from https://www.hpbonline.org/article/S1365-182X(16)31336-3/pdf

[110] Lee J, Miller P, Kermani R, et al. Gallbladder damage control: Compromised procedure for compromised patients. Surgical Endoscopy. 2012;**26**:2779-2783. DOI: 10.1007/s00464-012-2278-4

[111] Kutcher ME, Sperry JL, Rosengart MR, et al. Surgical rescue: The next pillar of acute care surgery. Journal of Trauma and Acute Care Surgery. 2017;**82**:280-286. DOI: 10.1097/TA.0000000000001312

[112] Függer R. Challenging situations in cholecystectomy and strategies to overcome them. European Surgery. 2021;**53**:106-113. DOI: 10.1007/s10353-020-00687-4

[113] Tan JR, Lunevicius R. Cholecystoappendiceal fistula associated with xanthogranulomatous cholecystitis. BMJ Case Reports. 2024;**17**:e260954. DOI: 10.1136/bcr-2024-260954

[114] Zino S, Mirza A, Nassar MK, et al. A difficulty grading system for laparoscopic cholecystectomy. In: ASGBI International Surgical Congress 2014, April 30-May 2, Harrogate, United Kingdom. ePostersLive® by SciGen® Technologies S.A. Available from: https://www.epostersonline.com/asgbi2014/node/3459

[115] Griffiths EA, Hodson J, Vohra RS, et al. Utilisation of an operative difficulty grading scale for laparoscopic cholecystectomy. Surgical Endoscopy. 2019;**33**:110-121. DOI: 10.1007/s00464-018-6281-2. Erratum in: Surgical Endoscopy. 2018 Aug 22. Erratum in: Surg Endosc 2023;37:2415

[116] Nassar AHM, Ng HJ, Wysocki AP, et al. Achieving the critical view of safety in the difficult laparoscopic cholecystectomy: A prospective study of predictors of failure. Surgical Endoscopy. 2021;**35**:6039-6047. DOI: 10.1007/s00464-020-08093-3

[117] Peponis T, Eskesen TG, Mesar T, et al. Bile spillage as a risk factor for surgical site infection after laparoscopic cholecystectomy: A prospective study of 1,001 patients. Journal of the American College of Surgeons. 2018;**226**:1030-1035. DOI: 10.1016/j.jamcollsurg.2017.11.025

[118] Edergren Å, Sandblom G, Agustsson T, Jaafar G. Intraoperative gallbladder perforation and risk of postoperative abscess with or without antibiotics: National cohort study of more than 108 000 cholecystectomies. British Journal of Surgery. 2023;**110**:896-900. DOI: 10.1093/bjs/znac351

[119] Hui TT, Giurgiu DI, Margulies DR, et al. Iatrogenic gallbladder perforation during laparoscopic cholecystectomy: Etiology and sequelae. The American Surgeon. 1999;**65**:944-948

[120] Strasberg SM, Bhalla S, Hammill CW. The pucker sign: An operative and radiological indicator of impending operative difficulty due to severe chronic contractive inflammation in cholecystectomy. Journal of Hepato-Biliary-Pancreatic Sciences. 2018;**25**:455-459. DOI: 10.1002/jhbp.583

[121] Sabour AF, Matsushima K, Love BE, et al. Nationwide trends in the use of subtotal cholecystectomy for acute cholecystitis. Surgery. 2020;**167**:569-574. DOI: 10.1016/j.surg.2019.11.004

[122] Mesri M, Nzenwa I, Lunevicius R. Evaluating the patient and setting-specific factors that influenced the quality of informed consent in a

retrospective cohort of subtotal cholecystectomy patients. Journal of Laparoendoscopic & Advanced Surgical Techniques. Part A. 2021;**31**:77-84. DOI: 10.1089/lap.2020.0376

[123] Lunevicius R, Nzenwa IC, Mesri M. A nationwide analysis of gallbladder surgery in England between 2000 and 2019. Surgery. 2022;**171**:276-284. DOI: 10.1016/j.surg.2021.10.025

[124] Lunevicius R, Nzenwa IC, Mesri M. Supplemental data content to 'a nationwide analysis of gallbladder surgery in England between 2000 and 2019'. Mendeley Data. 2021. V1. DOI: 10.17632/gp9vfvs76n.1

[125] Lunevicius R. Cholecystectomy: Advances and issues. Journal of Clinical Medicine. 2022;**11**:3534. DOI: 10.3390/jcm11123534

[126] Buell JF, Cronin DC, Funaki B, et al. Devastating and fatal complications associated with combined vascular and bile duct injuries during cholecystectomy. Archives of Surgery. 2002;**137**:703-708; discussion 708-710. DOI: 10.1001/archsurg.137.6.703

[127] Strasberg SM. Error traps and vasculo-biliary injury in laparoscopic and open cholecystectomy. Journal of Hepato-Biliary-Pancreatic Surgery. 2008;**15**:284-292. DOI: 10.1007/s00534-007-1267-9

[128] Strasberg SM, Gouma DJ. 'Extreme' vasculobiliary injuries: Association with fundus-down cholecystectomy in severely inflamed gallbladders. HPB: The Official Journal of the International Hepato Pancreato Biliary Association. 2012;**14**:1-8. DOI: 10.1111/j.1477-2574.2011.00393.x

[129] Sarno G, Al-Sarira AA, Ghaneh P, et al. Cholecystectomy-related bile duct and vasculobiliary injuries. British Journal of Surgery. 2012;**99**:1129-1136. DOI: 10.1002/bjs.8806

[130] CholeS Study Group, West Midlands Research Collaborative. Population-based cohort study of outcomes following cholecystectomy for benign gallbladder diseases. British Journal of Surgery. 2016;**103**:1704-1715. DOI: 10.1002/bjs.10287. Erratum in: British Journal of Surgery. 2018;105:1222. DOI: 10.1002/bjs.10894